Five Point
Touch Therapy

"Pierre-Noël Delatte, M.D., has provided brilliant insight for those eager to explore self-healing through his five point acupressure therapy. He clearly demonstrates and explains how, given the right conditions, acupressure therapy can naturally boost immunity, biologically produce its own medicine, and heal the body."

KAM THYE CHOW,
FOUNDER OF LOTUS PALM SCHOOL AND
AUTHOR OF *ADVANCED THAI YOGA MASSAGE*

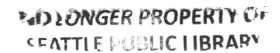

Five Point Touch Therapy

Acupressure for the Emotional Body

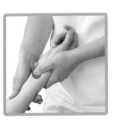
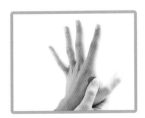
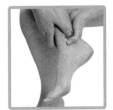
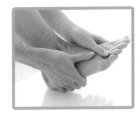

Pierre-Noël Delatte, M.D.

Translated by Brigitte Delatte

Healing Arts Press
Rochester, Vermont • Toronto, Canada

Healing Arts Press
One Park Street
Rochester, Vermont 05767
www.HealingArtsPress.com

Healing Arts Press is a division of Inner Traditions International

Originally published in French under the title *Cinq points, un point c'est tout!* by
  Guy Trédaniel Éditeur
First U.S. edition published in 2013 by Healing Arts Press

Note to the reader: *This book is intended as an informational guide. The remedies,
approaches, and techniques described herein are meant to supplement, and not to be a
substitute for, professional medical care or treatment. They should not be used to treat
a serious ailment without prior consultation with a qualified health care professional.*

Library of Congress Cataloging-in-Publication Data
Delatte, Pierre-Noël.
  [Cinq points, un point c'est tout! English]
  Five point touch therapy : acupressure for the emotional body / Pierre-Noël
Delatte, M.D. ; translated by Brigitte Delatte. — First U.S. edition.
    p. cm.
  Summary: "Simple and fast-acting self-treatment of emotional issues with
acupressure points"—Provided by publisher.
  Includes index.
  ISBN 978-1-59477-495-9 (pbk.) — ISBN 978-1-62055-135-6 (e-book)
  1. Acupuncture. 2. Acupuncture points. I. Title.
  RM184.D4513 2013
  615.8'92—dc23
                                                                2012031472

Printed and bound in the United States by Versa Press, Inc.

10 9 8 7 6 5 4 3 2 1

Text design and layout by Virginia Scott Bowman
This book was typeset in Garamond Premier Pro and Gill Sans with Avenir used
as the display typeface

To learn more about five point touch therapy or psycho-bio-acupressure (PBA), go
to **www.psycho-bio-acupressure.com**.

Contents

Introduction   1

1   What Is Five Point Touch Therapy or
Psycho-Bio-Acupressure (PBA)?   4

2   The Ten Most Commonly Used
Five Point PBA Circuits   19

3   Twelve Additional Five Point PBA Circuits   75

4   Combining the Circuits: Treatment Protocols   133

5   Glossary of Conditions and Recommended
Protocols   151

6   Five Golden Rules for Retaining Energy Balance   178

Conclusion   190

Appendix: The Evolution of Five Point Touch
Therapy   194

About the Author   196

Resources   197

Index   198

Introduction

During my decades-long practice as a general practitioner, I could not help but observe certain mind-boggling therapeutic results, which were not obtained by official medicine. Further, the mainstream mindset and official Cartesian perspective were at a loss when it came to explaining those baffling outcomes.

I decided to search for answers. Hoping for clarification, I took an interest in a large selection of therapies such as vibratory medicine, color therapy, chromo therapy, magnetism, crystals, essential oils, floral elixirs (the famous Bach essences as well as German Andrea Korte's elixirs), and so forth. I started to explore diverse alternative teachings such as a particular system devised by Doctor Patrick Véret, known as Nutripuncture, as well as mesotherapy and kinesiology. I learned with great interest about Mohammed Haddad's work on fractals and their successful use with certain types of cancer. In a word, I had a good look at many well-known and less-known systems that produce puzzling effects as yet unexplained by the general rational mindset.

For some reason, I felt I could not adhere to just one of the systems I learned about. So I decided not to limit myself to a single method, no matter how interesting it seemed. I did away with restricting boundaries and retained the systems with which I sensed a deeper harmony. My investigations, research, experiments, and selection of elements that could be amalgamated for the best results eventually produced a kind of melting pot. All this took me a long time, but my constant preoccupation and priority remained simplicity and rapidity of action to fight the enormity of the pain within and around us.

Over about fifteen years of extensive research I developed a five point touch therapy, which I have been sharing in my practice and the workshops I've been conducting for some time. This book has been written because of a promise I made to share what I have developed with an even wider circle. I made this promise to those who enrolled in the workshops and were asking for written words, and to those who regretted missing the opportunity to attend. I made this promise to those among my patients who were concerned about times when I could not be available and to those who asked me questions such as: "a member of my family who lives in France suffers from depression. Could you recommend somebody who does what you do?" To this, unhappily, I had no answer.

I'm definitely not a guru or a philosopher, but a little remark made by a friend, a Buddhist and a psychiatrist, has somehow made its way into my mind; he simply told me: "What has been given to you must be shared."

I have made this book as practical and accessible as possible, so that everyone who reads it can do what I do. My objective is to help my readers deal with unexpected life challenges as well as with everyday occurrences, such as helping a baby made restless and sleep-deprived by painful colic or fright of the dark, without having to drug her, or giving a parent the means to help her child overcome crippling exam jitters so that he can recover his full potential. Two five point circuits are all that it takes.

I honestly think that my colleagues (doctors, psychologists, sophrologists, osteopaths, acupuncturists, homeopaths, and so forth) could benefit from the addition of five point touch therapy to their existing training and knowledge; this is already the case for many physicians who have enrolled in the workshops I conduct.

In addition, five point touch therapy, which I also call psycho-bio-acupressure (PBA), can really help you reconnect with your personal accountability and take care of those endless incidents that inexorably add up and eventually ruin your day. A little discipline and five minutes are all you need.

In the pages that follow, you will first find, in chapter 1, a clear definition of exactly what five point touch therapy/psycho-bio-acupressure is, in theory and in practice, and a brief description of how I developed it. Chapters 2 and 3 provide detailed descriptions of the twenty-two five point circuits used in PBA and the proper technique of their stimulation. Chapter 4 demonstrates the combining of the circuits into specific treatment protocols, followed in chapter 5 by a glossary of conditions and recommended protocols to alleviate them. Chapter 6 follows with an in-depth exploration of what I term the "five golden rules" for balancing energy, which help us to sustain the results of five point touch therapy. The appendix adds further detail about the evolution of five point touch therapy.

1

What Is Five Point Touch Therapy or Psycho-Bio-Acupressure (PBA)?

One cannot heal a part of the body as a part separate from the whole. The body cannot be healed as if it had nothing to do with the soul, and for the body and the spirit to be healthy, one has to take care of the spirit in the first place . . . Nowadays, it is a common mistake for the doctors to separate the soul from the body.

PLATO

Five point touch therapy or psycho-bio-acupressure is a simple, practical method, which has rapid results and is easily accessible and applicable to everyone:

✦ It is a *simple* method: it consists of the simultaneous pressure of five acupuncture points, which produces a "printed circuit" on the body. Each "printed circuit" specifically corresponds to a particular negative emotion that is being targeted. These circuits are then grouped into precisely defined protocols, selected according to the issue being dealt with.

✦ It is a *practical* method: it does not require any preparation whatsoever. It is discreet as well, for it can be used anywhere without attracting unwanted curiosity.

✦ It is a method with *rapid results*: a few minutes only are necessary to recover from extreme stress and to restore the means needed to manage it.

✦ It is a method that is *accessible to everyone*: no special knowledge is called for. Reading this book with attention as well as memorizing the different acupuncture points should be enough.

✦ Last but not least, besides being a very special self-acupressure method, PBA is *applicable to everyone*: it may be used to help other people, even children and babies.

Now just what does psycho-bio-acupressure (PBA) mean?

"P" stands for *psychological* because the stimulation of acupuncture points directly impacts our psychological state of mind. PBA successfully deals with temporary negative emotions (such as anger) as well as with more profound pathological issues (such as depressive states, chronic anxiety, or obsessions).

"B" stands for *bio,* which means "life," because controlling our psychological state means managing our vital energies, and because this action on our mind definitely resonates with our physical state. Psychosomatic diseases are alleviated in the process. Our life can be radically changed because our life force can be stimulated. Just as organic agriculture prevents the soil, water, and air from being poisoned through the abusive use of chemical pesticides, biotherapies can prevent our bodies from being slowly poisoned through abusive use of psychotropic drugs. Instead, biotherapies enhance our body's natural healing abilities.

"A" stands for *acupressure,* which is the use of pressure to stimulate the ancient trigger points of acupuncture. While acupressure has been made known particularly through shiatsu, PBA uses a different and very specific technique involving the simultaneous application of five points.

The technique of five point touch therapy or PBA allows:

✦ *The instantaneous management of temporary emotions* in order to handle different types of situations ranging from common anxiety before an exam to a panic attack before boarding a plane. It can also be of a great help in the management of tragic situations such as a loss; although obviously PBA cannot magically erase the grief, it offers the possibility of coping with a crisis situation as efficiently as possible given the circumstances.

✦ *The treatment of lasting emotional states,* which are occasionally deeply anchored in the mind, and are prone to induce serious pathological conditions such as depression, obsessions, or chronic anxiety.

✦ *The alleviation of the emotional component of many psychosomatic disorders or illnesses,* such as eczema, stomach ulcers, or colitis and, as a consequence, the facilitated healing of those disorders.

Some Examples of the Use of Five Point Touch Therapy: Case Studies

Five point touch therapy is of a great help in the majority of upsetting and even traumatic situations, which can be demonstrated by a few case studies taken from my practice. Let me begin with a case of a sudden loss, precipitating a major crisis in a person who came to me for treatment.

CASE STUDY

PBA for Grief

Martha had recently lost her husband, who unexpectedly succumbed to a cerebral cardiovascular accident. Martha did her best to look strong, though she visibly had no strength and courage left; she was food- and sleep-deprived and found herself in tears the minute she was left by herself.

I selected the Distress Protocol (which will be described in detail in chapter 4); that is, through acupressure, I "printed" on her body the special circuits that take care of, in this sequence, negativity, depression, panic, excessive emotion, and the aftereffects of a trauma. I ended the session with the circuit that restores general energetic balance.

As early as the third circuit—about five minutes into the session—I observed that Martha was clearly relaxing. It did not take her long to confirm: "This is amazing; that terrible tension inside my head is gone." At the end of circuit number four, she said: "I feel as though that weight that suffocated me since my husband's death is fading away; now I can breathe again." At the end of the session, she acknowledged how radically better she felt: "I can't believe how much quieter and more relaxed I am now."

Of course, Martha's road to complete healing was still long, her grief was still there, and her difficulties had not gone away, but because she had recovered her energetic potential, she found herself in a position to deal more capably with her sorrow and her circumstances. I taught her the PBA circuits she needed, so that she could use them by herself whenever she felt she required them.

Temporarily disturbing emotions can be wiped away so that the skill to deal with the challenge at hand can resurface, as is shown by the following case.

CASE STUDY
Intense Fear of Driving Test

For a very long time, twenty-four-year-old Virginia had attempted to obtain her driver's license. She seemed to be a natural during her lessons, but she could not cope with the pressure of the test itself and was unable to keep her emotions in check: her heart painfully pounded, stomach burns instantly developed, her vision suddenly blurred, and, invariably, she ended in driving through a red light. This was the usual pattern of her driving tests, which she had tried and failed thirteen-odd times, which seems unbelievable yet is true.

Virginia was desperate to have her own car because her future job required it; her situation was clear: no driver's license, no job. A whole year had already gone by, and the more she tried, the less confident she felt. Her partner was starting to be critical of her alarming lack of self-control and determination. She had tried everything that might help, but found that she had no means to cope with her panic attacks. Neither prescribed medication (beta blockers) nor homeopathy had worked on her. She came to consult me without high hopes, but rather to please a friend who had warmly recommended me.

I concentrated on her pulse in order to feel her emotional state. I restored her energy through PBA circuits I'll introduce later in this book. Then, I taught her how to do three specific circuits herself: the first one dealt with panic, the second encouraged and improved all forms of expression, and the third one restored her energetic balance.

Some days later, a triumphant phone call let me know that she had passed her test and that she had hardly recognized her usual self; her new state of relaxation had allowed her to respond even to a tricky situation, which would have totally destabilized her at other times.

Examples like this one are daily occurrences in my practice. The circuits benefit a very broad range of different cases: a lawyer can stimulate certain PBA circuits before pleading a case; likewise, a comedian can deal with his stage fright fifteen minutes before going on stage.

Students find it possible to get rid of their exam jitters. Easily-learned five point circuits can take care of all those common emotions, which impact very negatively on our daily lives.

In addition to being of great help during emergency situations, the contribution of five point touch therapy to the resolution of chronic problems is also considerable, especially when a chronic issue threatens to become, or has already become, pathological. Let us take the example of Jack, who had been relocated (from France to New Caledonia) because of his firm's interests.

CASE STUDY
Separation from Family

For two years, Jack had to leave his young family behind. His wife had her own job and the children needed to stay at their old school. As they say in New Caledonia, Jack was a "geographical single person," who suffered very much from solitude. When he consulted me, he had made no new friends and liquor was becoming an easy as well as dangerous after-work habit. Jack was bored out of his wits and on his way to depression.

I applied the Depression Protocol, which really worked and helped for some weeks. Then he had a relapse, as his situation remained unchanged and the same causes produced the same effects because of his latent negative thinking, Not wanting to be on Prozac as suggested by his GP, he consulted me again. I recommended that he enroll in one of my workshops so that he could learn the different circuits that could help him avoid depression. I knew that my treatments could only bring temporary relief for a problem such as his, which was tied to a particular time span. When he came to see me again about a month after the workshop, he told me the following anecdote: "After the workshop, I felt so great that I neglected to work on myself every morning as you recommended. I just thought I felt fine. Then, a fortnight ago, my boss invited me to his place; I really did not feel like going, but I had to, so I did the circuits, especially the one against depression. I was amazed to find that I did enjoy myself that evening. Also, the next day, I still felt full of energy and retained a sense of purpose; I really felt positive and time just flew by, whereas a working day usually looks endless to me. Well, this helped me to realize that I just have to spend a little time every morning to do my circuits and that this little amount of time guarantees me a much more relaxed day." Naturally, Jack's situation had not changed, but he had gained the means to avoid depression and to wait serenely for the moment when he could be reunited with his little family.

PBA helps with children and even babies as well, as the following example demonstrates.

CASE STUDY
Infant Panic

Eight-month-old Kevin had not been able to sleep since he was born. The whole family was exhausted, and the couple was on the verge of separation; each night, the father and the mother had to take turns holding baby Kevin, but no sooner was the child put back into his own bed than the cries started afresh.

Different approaches to the problem had been tried, as well as the one suggested by the pediatrician (let the baby cry and wait till he stops out of exhaustion). Nothing worked and Kevin cried his little heart out; it seemed as if nothing could be done. Homeopathy did not have results, though some chemical drugs did, but then, the parents rejected the idea of putting chemicals inside Kevin's system.

When I saw the baby for the first time, I started to inquire about the pregnancy and the delivery. Kevin's mother had previously lost her first baby after six months of pregnancy, and this accident had made her highly sensitive to a potential repetition of this first experience: she felt extremely anxious and had to stop working early in her pregnancy precisely because of this high anxiety. The delivery itself had been a disaster: eight days after he was due, Kevin gave no indication whatsoever of wanting to be born; meanwhile, the placenta was showing signs of growing old. Labor had to be induced and contractions were difficult and painful. In the end, forceps had to be used. As Kevin's mother said: "It appeared as if the baby was just rejecting the very idea of being born."

Actually this case is extremely common: the baby is simply terrified. In this case, baby Kevin had felt and absorbed his mother's deep anxiety while he was in her womb; he had also strongly perceived her terror of losing him when the date of delivery was approaching. Finally, the use of forceps most probably appeared to him as an act of aggression. No wonder then that Kevin was afraid to fall asleep.

We know that one of the major fears of our forefathers was to be attacked during their sleep and that this fear remains encoded within the most primitive part of our brain. This fear is as ancient as the beginnings of humanity. Even at this stage of our evolution, our unconscious mind considers sleeping as a potentially dangerous loss of control of our environment. According to its logic, it also considers staying awake as the best way to avoid any latent danger in time of high anxiety; this becomes a kind of reflex. Incidentally, do not we say "fall" in love, "fall" asleep, and "fall" ill? These situations reflect our major fears of losing control (of our heart, of our environment, of our body). Kevin was obviously in a state of panic and it made sense that he simply could not "fall" asleep.

I applied the five point circuits that take care of the state of panic and the aftereffects of a trauma; I also selected the ones that restore the energetic system. To be on the safe side, I also did the circuit related to colic (fear often expresses itself through colic). That night, little Kevin slept like an angel for the first time.

His parents called me the next morning and half-jokingly asked me if I was a magician. I'm not of course; the case of Kevin just required the right questions, some common sense, and application of the appropriate five point circuits to solve the problem at its source.

As these case studies make clear, PBA can prevent an aggravation of our emotional state when it is applied with vigilance and discipline as soon as the first signs of discomfort appear. At the same time, it certainly does not limit itself to temporary incidents. When used preventively, it can prevent a situation from degenerating into chaos; in that respect, we have to stay humble and bear in mind that the mind-body connection is a reality.

Any lasting psychological or emotional disturbance is capable of leading to physical disorders. Five point touch therapy makes it possible for us to regain control of the situation; the sooner we make use of it, the more we will protect and enhance our health. It would definitely be a good idea to adopt the Eastern approach to illness that consists in giving priority to preventive medicine rather than healing problems that already exist.

I personally live a very hectic life, which many would consider exhausting. I travel year round so as to share PBA through seminars and workshops (this means constant plane and train travels, staying in hotels, and working all weekdays and weekends). As well as working in Europe and different regions of the world, I regularly fly back to Australia where my family lives. Still, I feel younger than I did ten years ago.

How Five Point Touch Therapy Works

In order to understand how five point touch therapy/PBA works, we need to briefly explore the concept of *vital energy*.

Throughout history, cultures all over the world have acknowledged the existence of a universal energy, a force present in the whole universe including the human body; it has been given many names, such as *prana* in India, *chi* or *ki* in the Far East, *chula* in some shamanistic traditions and *animus* in Latin. Invisible like air, vital energy has a deep influence on our health and our comfort. Not only does it have an impact on our physical health and on our survival, it is also responsible for our mental and emotional balance.

Basically, physical health is good as long as vital energy is well balanced and allowed a free flow; when energy is blocked or unbalanced, troubles emerge, which may grow into diseases.

Let us keep in mind that all matter, regardless of how dense it may be, is made of energy. It is constituted of atoms, protons, and electrons, which vibrate together at different frequencies. We inhabit the electromagnetic field of the earth, and are surrounded by waves, from the low frequency of radio waves at one end of the spectrum to the high frequency cosmic rays at the other end. Absolutely everything in the universe is constituted of energy, which grows denser and starts to vibrate at a lower frequency when it becomes matter. This energy field is an immense grid that encompasses everything. This is where we live, all of us. This is what connects us all.

We humans are also energetic phenomena. We operate in our own energy fields. Our vital energy radiates all around our physical body (this "aura" can be seen by some); it enters and leaves our body through energy centers called *chakras* and circulates along corridors of energy called meridians or *nadis*.

Health problems manifest themselves when energy is congested or when its stimulation is too high or too low. Health is good when different levels of energy within and around the body are well balanced, when a condition of equilibrium prevails. One of the most ancient of healing systems, acupuncture, involves the insertion of fine needles into specific points of the body in order to regulate the flow of energy through the meridians.

Chinese medicine acknowledges two complementary energies, yin and yang, which together constitute the chi or vital energy. Certain organs are yin, the liver, for example, while others are yang, such as the stomach. In the same way, there are six yin meridians and six yang meridians. There are about 365 acupuncture points along those meridians where the vital energy is concentrated. The insertion of acupuncture needles into the skin at these specific points allows the stimulation or the reduction of the flow of energy through the meridians; this influences the quality of energy that reaches the organs and rebalances the way they work. A proper circulation of energy provides us with a sense of harmony.

For the skeptics, let us mention here that, although these famous meridians have no anatomical support, their existence has recently been demonstrated by Western science: the variations of the beta radiations along their course have been recorded and mapped out on meditating yogis.

In the beginning I was inspired by a "five point acupuncture" technique, which is taught in Australia and in different parts of the world. In France, Doctor Patrick Véret was a precursor in this field. Rather than considering the energy of an isolated acupuncture point, the initial reasoning was to stimulate five points at the same time, so as to produce a printed circuit on the body. Derived from the original energy that circulates within the meridians, a specific energy would start flowing within the circuit. Each specific circuit (constituted of five points) was seen to correspond to a particular issue.

I was taught this particular technique about eighteen years ago, and I decided to use it in my practice. I learned certain circuits through Dr. Véret's writings and others from other sources. My purpose at that time was to use the circuits in order to deal with physical disorders such as hypertension, sinusitis, or sciatica. However, the results I obtained were a bit surprising. My patients did not seem to draw any benefit from the circuits, at least not on the physical level. Unexpectedly, their psychological reactions proved unanimous: they reported feeling better, more relaxed, with their usual stress gone.

After giving this a lot of thought, I carefully experimented for a long time. Eventually I could not help but draw the unanticipated yet crystal-clear conclusion that those circuits produced an unknown psychological impact. Let me now try to explain it to you in simple terms and by using a comparison. Certain aspects of our brain and of our body (which depends on our brain) share similarities with a computer; if the computer is not connected to the right voltage, or if its battery is low, certain programs just stop working. The same happens with our brain: as soon as it ceases to be correctly fed, certain "programs" stop working, making us unable to handle the situations that come our way. This comparison with a computer is obviously just a useful metaphor (the brain is not a machine), but this metaphor makes the whole process easy to understand.

The energy that goes to our brain and feeds it originates in large part from our thoughts. *Thought is pure energy:* the full meaning of this concept as well as its implications is very important to understanding five point touch therapy/psycho-bio-acupressure. Thought is an energetic phenomenon and its impact is not to be underestimated. This is a concept made familiar by quantum physics.

Of course, we receive energies from our metabolism (hence the importance of trace elements), as well as from our cosmic and telluric environment. *However, the thought-induced energies are the ones that have a major impact on our brain (and are liable to disturb it).* This is also an observable reality. Each of us experiences a glimpse of this every day.

Just observing the way we feel when we are speaking with an angry person makes us aware that we are dealing with fields of energy: whatever efforts that person makes to conceal his strong feelings of anger, we just *know* it, we feel the energy that emanates from him; that energy originates from his thoughts and radiates powerfully. However hard the angry person endeavors to appear collected, we pick up on that energy of anger. On the contrary, the energy of love coming from a person in love is warm, powerful, and beautiful.

Unsurprisingly, each time we charge our brain with negativity, our "voltage" decreases, and this is what makes us unable to cope with our challenges. The more we are charged with negative energies, the more we disturb the way we function, *until we finally switch to different energetic systems,* which can be systems of depression or panic. The particular incident that triggers our destructive emotion might be so unbearable that it makes us lose control or "blow our fuses," and this is how a "scar" is produced in our energetic system. Such "scars" have enduring effects on our future.

To come back to our comparison with electricity, let us just say that if a number of fuses, which have blown in your home, are not fixed, the small appliances that correspond to them will just stop working. This situation will last forever if nothing is done. This much is very clear. The same process occurs with our brain. However, just as we can repair the fuses in our homes, we have the possibility of restoring balance to our energies.

This is where five point touch therapy comes in. By stimulating certain specific PBA circuits, an energy antidote will start flowing; *in a matter of minutes, our energy will be restored; relief will be instantaneous.*

The Birth of
Five Point Touch Therapy

When I started to work with five point circuits, I employed needles as I had been trained to do, although I realized at an early stage that certain points could be very sensitive and therefore induce an energy that quite possibly interfered with the efficiency of the circuits. Also I wanted to take care of babies, and needles were obviously not the solution there.

A brief incident changed all that: one day, while strolling in Chinatown in Sydney, I began on an impulse to explain my dilemma to a needle salesman; he suggested that I give his patches a try. Those patches contained tiny balls capable of activating the points; they were used occasionally by Asian people to get rid of migraines. So I gave those patches a try without being really convinced of their efficiency. To my amazement, they worked.

How they worked is related to the fact that an acupuncture point may be impacted in two different ways: stimulating (toning up) its energy or diminishing (scattering) its surplus energy. Stimulation of the points can be obtained through needles, heat, or manual pressure.

✦ In the case of *needles,* once the needle has been inserted, it has to be rotated clockwise in order to tone up; another way is to use a gold needle. To scatter, the needle is rotated in a counterclockwise movement; alternatively, a silver needle is used.

✦ *Heat* can also be used to tone: the most common techniques are little sticks of burning wormwood, called *moxa,* or light obtained through optic fibers.

✦ Finally, *stimulation* can be caused by manual pressure, which is how the patches worked.

In the work I was doing, the goal was to stimulate rather than scatter energy. For this, the patches offered a pain-free solution. For months, I used them in five point circuits on babies and children with great success. Then, one day, a patient whose baby I had taken care of confessed that she would like to have a PBA session but that she had a phobia of needles. At that time, I was only using patches with babies and children; for some reason, I still believed in the superiority of needles. However, I sensed a new opportunity and decided in this case to work with patches. The results of the session went far beyond my expectations and helped me to make up my mind that from then on, I would employ patches exclusively, whatever the age of my patient.

The second step in the development of my original method was taken during another trip abroad, when I was asked to help a depressed young woman; she was a guest of friends who were well aware of the positive results I had been getting. I could not possibly refuse, although having no patches at my disposal made me uncomfortable. I had never before experimented with manual pressure and I had not the slightest idea if the printed circuit could work without patches. However, I really wanted to respond to my friends' request, so I had no other choice than to try with my fingers. I firmly pressed on the five points. *The result was absolutely impressive and almost instantaneous.* In just a few minutes, the young woman reported that she felt totally relaxed and that the heavy weight she had had on her chest was gone.

As I experimented with various circuits over a long period of time, I eventually selected and modified twenty-two that demonstrated the most usefulness in relation to our mental functioning. Some circuits deal with the elimination of energies of depression, panic, hyper-emotionality, negativity, or obsession. Others positively charge all our energy centers or wipe away ancient scars imprinted in our energetic system by past distressing episodes of our lives.

Eventually I grouped the definitive circuits into very precise protocols, each one targeting a specific psychological situation. These protocols aid us in coping with a destabilizing situation, precisely without . . . destabilizing us. (Please see the appendix for a more detailed description of my development of five point touch therapy.)

Slowly but surely I realized that if no needles or patches were needed, five point touch therapy could be taught as a self-help method. The foundation of inner harmony is a healthy energetic system, which PBA makes possible for anyone. I started with my patients in my practice, before organizing and conducting little workshops, which soon became quite popular. While just ten minutes devoted to PBA at the beginning of each new day is all that is needed, knowledge of the circuits, presented in the next two chapters, is a necessary foundation.

2
The Ten Most Commonly Used Five Point PBA Circuits

Psycho-bio-acupressure relies on nine principal five point circuits to clear negative energies and restore a positive charge. They are the most commonly used, so it is essential to be familiar with them. These circuits, which I teach during my workshops, are quite easy to memorize. I have added a tenth one, which is not as regularly used. Despite its relative rarity of application, it may be extremely useful in unblocking certain situations, which is the reason why I include it here.

First, let's talk about the application technique, which pertains to all of the circuits. The first step is to learn the precise location on the body of the five points of each circuit.

Locating the Points

For each PBA point listed in this book, four guides to its location are given:

1. For readers who are familiar with acupuncture or shiatsu, each point is listed with its identification number as indicated in the standard referencing system used by professionals.

19

2. Each is described using standard anatomical terms for body parts and locations.

3. A visual illustration of each point on the body is given.

4. Instructions for locating the point accompany the illustrations.

Despite the accuracy of the illustrations, you may feel some uncertainty because the point locations vary slightly depending on the person. If you do not feel confident, don't hesitate to explore the area around the point. Place your thumb, forefinger, or index finger (depending on what you feel most comfortable with) on the spot depicted on the illustration. Your other fingers are not strong enough to awaken any sensitivity. While keeping your finger on the depicted spot, press harder, a bit on the right hand side, a bit on the left, slightly above and slightly below, until you hit a more sensitive zone: this is the point you want. When this is done, maintain the pressure, firmly and steadily, but not painfully, for about five seconds.

Do not worry if you perceive a slight difference between the location of the most sensitive point you have identified and the location of its correspondent point as depicted in the standard referencing system. For the lay reader, it will be most convenient and sufficient to use the last two location guides—the visual illustrations and instructions. However, the other numbers and terms are provided for ready access for professionals. The lay reader may also find it helpful to refer to the following definitions of standard anatomical location terms:

Distal: situated away from the center of the body or from the point of attachment

Proximal: situated nearer to the center of the body or the point of attachment

Medial: situated near the midline of the body or the midline of an organ

Lateral: the opposite of medial; near or on the side or sides of the body

Dorsal: toward the top, toward the upper side or the back of the body

Ventral: toward the underside of the body

In addition, you may find the following conversion table to be helpful.

> **Converting Centimeters to Inches**
>
> **1 cm = 0.39 in**

Application Technique

Once you have located each of the five points in a given circuit, the goal is to awaken their sensitivity through pressure. *The technique consists in applying a firm manual pressure for a few seconds to each of the five points in turn, then, without pausing, applying a second and third pressure, a bit quicker.* The pressure has to be firm but not painful; a balance has to be found. Sensitivity needs to be felt in all five points at once. If you are not feeling one of the acupressure points after you have finished the circuit, do not hesitate to apply fresh pressure to it, perhaps for a little longer time.

The objective is to stimulate the five points sufficiently so that the tissues will keep the memory of the pressure. In other words, after we have stopped pressing on the five points, we (or our patient) should feel that the pressure lingers in all five points for a few moments. This is crucial: we don't press hard enough to cause pain (but almost); at the same time we have to make sure the pressure is firm enough for the tissues to keep the memory of it. This is how a "printed circuit" is produced. The pressure causes the energy we want to activate to begin flowing into the circuit.

Let's suppose, for example, that you want to stimulate point 4 of the circuit against depression.

Separate your left thumb from your left index finger. Place your right thumb right into the angle that has been produced. Press firmly. Slowly rotate clockwise till you hit a more sensitive zone: here is the acupressure point you want. Remember this special sensitivity: this is what you will be looking for when searching for any of the other acupressure points detailed in this book.

Nonetheless, if you don't find this sensitive zone, do not worry

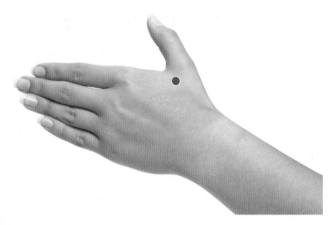

Point 4, depression circuit

too much, as it is possible that this specific area does not feel particularly special on you. Just press your finger on the point as shown on the sketch and apply a firm pressure. You can't go wrong because the surface of your finger largely covers the area you want to target.

Don't forget that a firm pressure does not mean a painful one: press firmly, dig deep to make sure you find this special sensitivity; the elasticity of your skin allows you to do that. *It is of the utmost importance that, after you have pressed upon the five points and closed your eyes to mentally check on them, you still feel the pressure lingering in each of the five: the five points have to remain activated together for a few seconds for the circuit to start working and become effective.*

Also do not forget to remove your watch (because of the batteries) and to empty your pockets of items such as mobile phones, remote controls, and magnetic bracelets or necklaces, as these objects could interfere with the action of PBA. In the same way, if you are working on somebody else, ensure that they remove all such objects.

When you are working on someone else it is also important to mentally build a "neutral shield" (see the fourth golden rule in chapter 6) to protect yourself against negative energies, and to wash your hands carefully once the session is over. It does not serve anyone if you become charged with energies that are not your own.

Overcoming Self-Sabotage

It may appear safe to assume that, once we have made up our mind to use PBA in order to work on ourselves, we are fully aware of what we are doing and that our willpower is strong because we really have the intention of getting better. Or, if a patient consults us for the express purpose of improving well-being, it seems as though that should be the case.

However, self-sabotage can manifest in any of us, when a conflict arises between the conscious and the unconscious. Consciously, the patient may indeed want to recover, but her unconscious mind may not. Without realizing it, she may be drawing secondary gains from an unpleasant situation. For example, a woman suffering from a severe depression may honestly believe that she really wants to get better, whereas her unconscious wishes for this situation to endure, as family and friends are concerned and take care of her. Somehow being the center of attention is a benefit of some sort.

This concept has been well explained by Roger Callahan in his remarkable book *Five Minute Phobia Cure* (Enterprise Publishing, 1985) in which he discusses the concept of "psychological inversion." Other scientists mention this notion as well, such as Doctor Patrick Véret in his work *La médecine cosmogénétique ou l'Energo-médecine* (Cosmogenetic Medicine or Energetic Medicine) (Editions du Rocher, 1991) or Michel Dogna in his impressive book *Manuel du nouveau thérapeute* (Manual for the New Therapist) (Editions Guy Trédaniel, 2012).

Both Véret and Dogna also present the value of what I term "muscle testing" to determine if such self-sabotage is present. Doctor Jean Elmiger from Lausanne (Switzerland) develops this notion as well in his book *Rediscovering Real Medicine: The New Horizons of Homeopathy* (Element Books, 1998). Doctor Véret called it "neuromuscular testing" and Michel Dogna "universal bio testing." Whatever name it is given, the important thing is that it really works. It can be used to check whether the vibrations of a chemical affect our system in a negative way. In the situation that interests us here, it allows us to check on a person's real desire to recover, and to remedy the situation instantly in case of self-sabotage.

It is a very simple procedure. First ask the patient to keep his left arm in a horizontal position, and tell him to prevent you from lowering it. Put your own left hand on his right shoulder to help him keep his balance, then, using your right hand, press upon his left wrist as hard as possible in order to test his strength until his resistance limit is reached. Now ask your patient to think or, even better, to say aloud, that he wants to get better (or to stop being afraid, or to lose weight, etc.) and repeat the pressure upon his wrist. If the patient's intention is strong and if his desire to recover is genuine, then his strength will remain the same. But with self-sabotage, the strength to resist disappears and the arm just drops (see illustration).

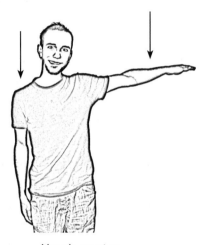

Muscle testing

If the arm drops, make the patient close his fist and, using the point of your second finger, tap 35 times on the fold below the fifth finger as shown in the facing illustration.

Repeat the operation on the other closed fist. When this is done, repeat the muscle test and ask the patient to say again that he wants to get better and you'll observe this time that the patient's arm keeps its full strength. This process is a very simple application of kinesiology (see box on page 26) that easily gets rid of self-sabotage. The effect will probably be relatively short-lived, yet this will be enough for the circuits to work without being threatened by an "inner saboteur."

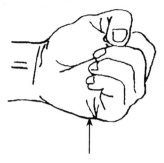

Tap the fold below the fifth finger.

The principle of this muscle testing is simple: as our thoughts are an energetic phenomenon, if a thought perturbs us (such as thinking we want to get better whereas our unconscious does not), it produces a parasitic energy that disrupts our nerve impulses; as a consequence, we lose our muscular strength. When the thought is no longer disturbing, we regain our full strength. This is true for any kind of thought: a thought that is not in harmony with us and disturbs us, affects our endurance.

Note: If, for some reason (pain, arthritis) you find that you can't use the shoulder testing, you can use any other muscular group (such as thwarted flexion of the elbow, opening of the closed fist, stretching of a bent leg). Any action that allows the measurement of the original muscular strength and its subsequent deficit in case of self-sabotage can be used.

An extra benefit of this testing is that you can use it on yourself if you don't feel very sure about your current state of mind. It is very hard to have sufficient objectivity and lucidity to be the judge of how you really feel, so if you suspect a little anxiety, negativity, or even depression lurking in you, you can ask somebody to help you by applying a firm pressure on your arm while you think: "I'm in a negative frame of mind." In case of a negative answer, your arm drops, meaning that you are *not* negative and do not expressly need the circuit. In the same way, when you want to know what the person you are helping really needs, you may use this testing, which cannot go wrong.

Note about Kinesiology

In the sixties, an American chiropractor, George Goodheart, noticed that muscles can be fortified when other apparently unrelated parts of the body are massaged or pressed upon. This apparent oddity is possible because the body is an integral whole and because all major organs and systems are interconnected through energy circuits. An excess energy or an energy that is blocked inside the energy canals may produce a weakness in the corresponding organ and can be detected in the related muscle. For example, the quadriceps is connected to the small intestine; in a case of lactose intolerance, if one drinks a glass of milk, the intolerance will be felt not only in the intestine but in the quadriceps as well. In testing the strength of the different muscles, a specialist in kinesiology can source the cause of the problem.

Kinesiology considers health as constituted of three aspects in a "health triangle": structural (physical), mental, and chemical. The patient is asked to resist a certain pressure on one limb. The energy circuit of the muscle turns off when a meridian or a particular organ is imbalanced.

Three kinds of "challenges" help to determine what is wrong:

1. Physical challenge
2. Chemical challenge: chemical substances or homeopathic dilutions are directly placed on the tongue or on the skin.
3. Mental challenge: the patient is asked to concentrate on certain thoughts or sentiments and the difference in his or her muscular resistance strength is tested. (Many chronic diseases have a strong emotional foundation, and the hidden cause of the issue is revealed in this way.) The mental challenge is the one used to search for self-sabotage.

Circuit 1

Against Depression

Basically, depression is characterized by a certain number of cardinal signs:

> *Exhaustion:* an intense tiredness manifests itself, particularly in the morning. The person gets up already exhausted. Feeling tired in the evening is clearly normal, whereas feeling tired in the morning is definitely not. If getting out of bed requires a superhuman effort, this may be a sign of depression.
>
> *Insomnia:* difficulty in going to sleep or sleep interrupted by long periods of wakefulness or nightmares. In a word, sleep is never refreshing. Sometimes, instead of insomnia, the depressed person might seek refuge in sleep and sleep an excessive amount of time (but this is more rare).
>
> *Apathy:* absence or impairment of willpower. The person is incapable of putting anything into action and is lacking energy to a point that he cuts himself off from the usual daily life. Total absence of feelings and initiative has replaced everything else.
>
> *Anorexia:* of course, it's hard to feel hungry in this situation; an immense effort is required to feed oneself.
>
> *Bulimia or binge-purge syndrome:* this is more rare but may emerge to fill up the feeling of emptiness and insecurity within.
>
> *Morbid ideas:* if depression lasts too long, the will to live just disappears. The person is connected with the energy of non-existence and feels very sick and hypochondriac, often starts talking about suicide.

Be extremely cautious when dealing with this kind of case and seek professional advice.

I always start my workshops by teaching this circuit. Once everyone has understood how it works and has used it (participants work on each other), the tension that is inevitably present at the beginning of a workshop disappears as if by magic, and the group suddenly becomes harmonious and ready to work. This circuit can be used as well when you are feeling under pressure. Participants frequently reported later that doing this circuit at the end of a hard day really helped them to relax.

— Remember to press firmly for four or five seconds on each of the following five acupressure points before repeating the operation twice. The energy of depression will disappear in five minutes.

Point 1: Spleen 1 (Right)

(Medial side of the big toe, 0.1 cm proximal to the corner of the nail.)

Hold your right big toe and press firmly a little bit below the lower left corner of the nail.

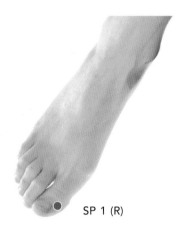

SP 1 (R)

Point 2: Triple Heater 15 (Left)

(In the depression midway between GB21 and SI13, in the suprascapular fossa.)

Put your right hand on the horizontal part of your left shoulder (top of trapezius). Your middle finger should be a little above the projecting part of your left shoulder blade (or scapula). The point you want should be right under the last phalanx of your middle finger. Press firmly; you should feel a more sensitive zone; if you don't, feel to the sides of the point until you feel more sensitivity. Do not hesitate to press firmly, as this point (like point 1) is not very sensitive and consequently hard to locate.

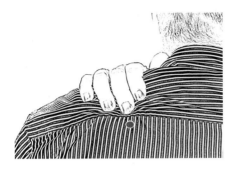

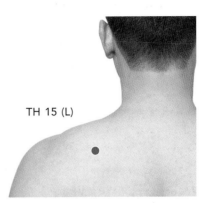

TH 15 (L)

Point 3: Lung 7 (Right)

(5 cm proximal to the most distal skin crease of the right wrist, proximal to the styloid of the radius in a depression between the bone and the tendons of brachioradialis and abductor pollicis longus.)

This is where your doctor usually feels your pulse. When you press, you will feel a little depression between the bone and the tendons responsible for the flexion of your hand. If you pay attention, you will feel the pulse beat there.

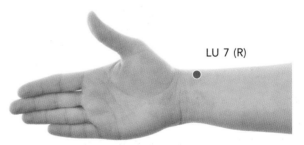

LU 7 (R)

Point 4: Large Intestine I4 (Left)

(Between the 1st and 2nd metacarpals of your left hand, on the radial aspect of the middle of the 2nd metacarpal bone, at the highest spot of the muscle when the thumb and index fingers are brought close together.)

Now look at the back of your left hand; separate your thumb from your index finger and place your right thumb just in the angle shown in the illustration, exactly at the point of the "V" formed by the two first metacarpal bones (the bones at the base of the thumb and index finger). Exert pressure. You'll observe a tender spot there.

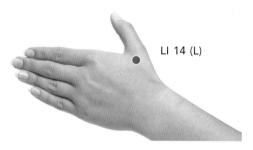

LI 14 (L)

Point 5: Conception Vessel 17

(In a depression on the midline, on the sternum, level with the 4th intercostal space.)

This point is right on the middle of the axis that connects the two nipples; it can be highly sensitive in very anxious persons. Alternatively, you may use the point situated five centimeters lower on the midline.

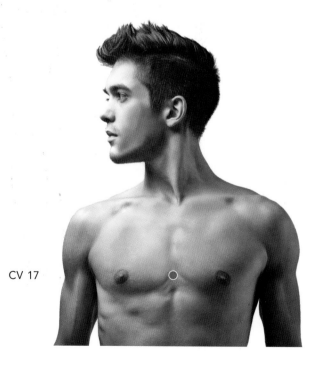

CV 17

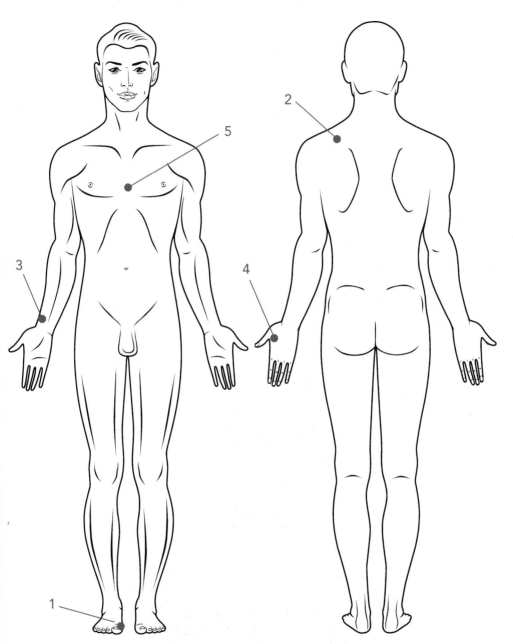

Circuit 1: Against Depression

Against Negativity

Negativity is easy to recognize: it is a state of mind where everything is perceived and experienced as negative and gloomy; being affected by negativity does not mean being really depressed, though negativity may well be a sign of depression if it lasts for too long.

Basically, being negative means invariably and exclusively seeing the negative side of events and people, and never their positive side; it means feeling antagonized and criticized all the time as well as exasperated by anything and everything around; negativity means seeing the empty half of the glass in all things; it means feeling separated from the rest of the world which is experienced as hostile.

Systematic doubt is part of negativity: you start your day feeling that nothing is going to work, you have stopped believing in anything, and you have the impression that you are just wasting your time. You are unable to visualize a horizon that could be free from the feeling of separation and loss. You begin to distrust your usual ethical values and whatever you used to believe in. You are blinded to insight and allow yourself to be overwhelmed by the cancer of systematic doubt. If we let doubt invade all aspects of our life, we are obviously in a negative state of mind and possibly on our way to depression.

This circuit is very effective in breaking negative patterns and helping us to regain a broader perspective. I use it myself often before going to work when I feel that it's going to be a hard day or when I'm honest with myself and recognize that I'm in a negative state of mind. It is extremely important, as it is part of practically every protocol we'll be studying a bit later. (These protocols made up of various circuits help us manage all the destructive emotions that weaken and destabilize us.)

Point 1: Spleen 6 (Left)

(On the internal side of the left ankle, 5 cm directly above the tip of the medial malleolus on the posterior border of the tibia.)

This point is situated on the inner side of the left ankle, about five centimeters above the prominence at the lower end of the tibia (larger lower leg bone). This point is often quite sensitive. If you work on yourself, place the little finger of your right hand on the bony projection: the point will be situated just under your index finger. Make sure you press upon the back edge of the tibia and *not* upon its front edge.

If you work on someone else, do as the sketch shows: put the little finger of your left hand on the bony projection; the point will be right under your index finger.

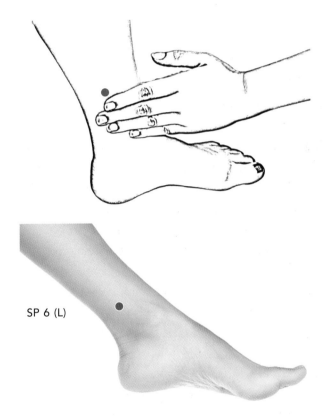

SP 6 (L)

Point 2: Large Intestine 4 (Right)

(Between the 1st and 2nd metacarpals of your right hand, on the radial aspect of the middle of the 2nd metacarpal bone, at the highest spot of the muscle when the thumb and index fingers are brought close together.)

This corresponds to point 4 in the circuit against depression, but this point is on the right hand. Separate your right thumb from your index finger and exert pressure right in the middle.

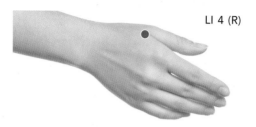

LI 4 (R)

Point 3: Special Point (Right Foot)

(Right foot, between the extensor tendons of the third and fourth toes, about 2 cm from their base.)

This point is on the back of the right foot, about two centimeters from the base of the toes, between the tendons of the third and fourth toes.

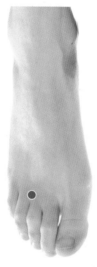

Point 4: Lung 7 (Left)

(5 cm proximal to the most distal skin crease of the left wrist, proximal to the styloid of the radius in a depression between the bone and the tendons of brachioradialis and abductor pollicis longus.)

This point corresponds to point 3 in circuit 1 against depression, only this time it is located on the left arm instead of the right. Located a little above the left wrist crease, it is where you feel your pulse.

LU 7 (L)

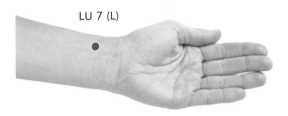

Point 5: Governing Vessel 23

(From the anterior hairline follow the sagittal line of the skull back until a depression is felt at the anterior fontanel.)

To find this point on yourself, look into a mirror as you follow the axis of the cranium back from your front hairline until you feel a little depression. This depression, which varies from individual to individual, corresponds to what remains of the anterior fontanel you had as a baby. This is exactly where you have to press.

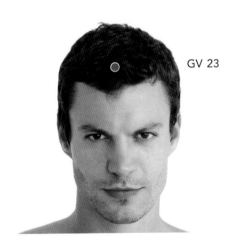

GV 23

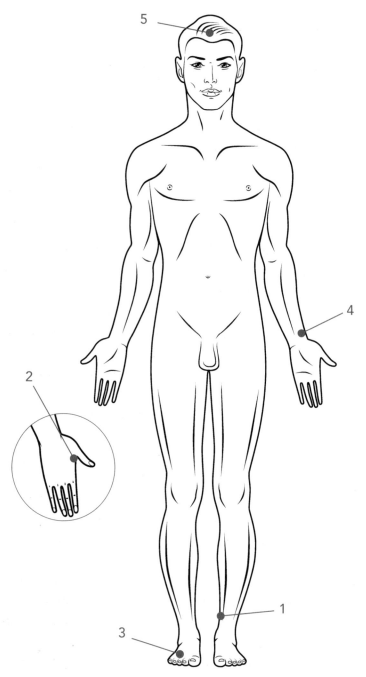

Circuit 2: Against Negativity

Against Fear, Anxiety, and Panic

This circuit applies to situations when the level of anxiety becomes unbearable and its impact physically difficult to bear.

Temporary fear (related to special circumstances): before a presentation or a job interview, before going on stage if you are an actor, or before a sport event if you are a participant, and so forth . . . No matter how well prepared you are, you are helpless and unproductive because of this fear.

Chronic anxiety: you are scared of everything without reason, feel that you are on the verge of constant disaster, and apprehensive about all phone calls; you constantly fear for family and friends as well as for your own wellness and professional status; in a word, your attitude denies you relaxation and pleasure and attests your lack of trust in the universe; you feel at the mercy of outside circumstances and let your anxiety grow into a generalized, unjustified, and pervasive fear that eventually dominates your entire existence.

Irrational panic: the kind that occurs before a car trip or plane travel.

Phobia (of spiders or snakes for example): Many of us have experienced this state of fear, which is bound to produce a psychosomatic reaction of some sort: shallow breathing, excessive sweating, extreme agitation, alarming heart rate, or the painful impression that your solar plexus is being crushed by a giant fist.

We have to find a way to diminish the pressure of anxiety; here again, PBA is there for us. It is a good idea to know this circuit by heart, as it is remarkably effective and is present in the majority of the protocols we'll be studying a little later in this book. The reasons for anxiety are numerous and liable to occur without warning, so doing this circuit on a regular basis is really helpful.

Point 1: Urinary Bladder 67 (Right)

(Lateral aspect of the right little toe, 0.1 cm proximal to the corner of the nail.)

To locate this point, firmly hold your right little toe between the thumb and the second finger of your right hand; carefully place your thumb upon the last phalanx, just before the corner of the nail and press firmly. This point is not very sensitive.

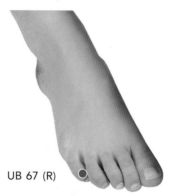

UB 67 (R)

Point 2: Kidney 1 (Right)

(On the sole of the foot, between the 2nd and 3rd metatarsal bones at the crease made by toe flexion at the MTP joints.)

Flex the toes of your right foot and press in the little depression that appears on the sole some five centimeters from the base of your toes. Make sure you remain on the center axis of the sole of your foot. This point is sensitive and corresponds to the beginning of the kidney meridian. Once you have identified this point, you won't forget it.

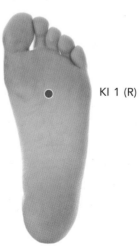

KI 1 (R)

Point 3: Conception Vessel 17

(In a depression on the midline, on the sternum, level with the 4th intercostal space.)

This point is located on the sternum exactly between the nipples, on the median axis of the chest. Alternatively, you can use the point situated about five centimeters lower on the same axis.

This is the same as point 5 in circuit 1 against depression.

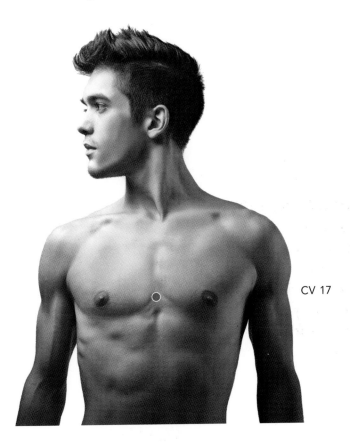

CV 17

Point 4: Triple Heater 5 (Left)

(5 cm proximal to the dorsal wrist crease between the radius and ulna, close to the radial bone.)

Place your left hand upon your right shoulder; firmly hold your shoulder: now, place your left arm close against your chest. This enables you to uncross the two bones of your left forearm. Now, with the first three fingers of your right hand, press right between the two bones (about five centimeters from the base of your wrist). This is about where a watch usually rests.

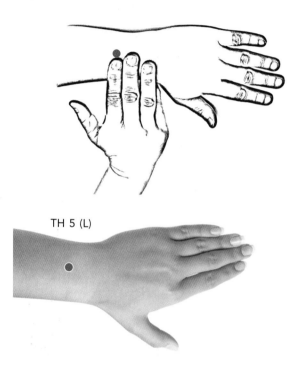

TH 5 (L)

Point 5: Spleen 1 (Left)

(Medial side of the great toe, 0.1 cm proximal to the corner of the nail.)

This is the symmetrical point of point 1 in circuit 1 against depression.

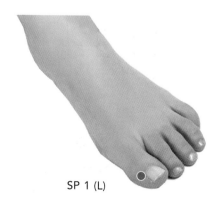

SP 1 (L)

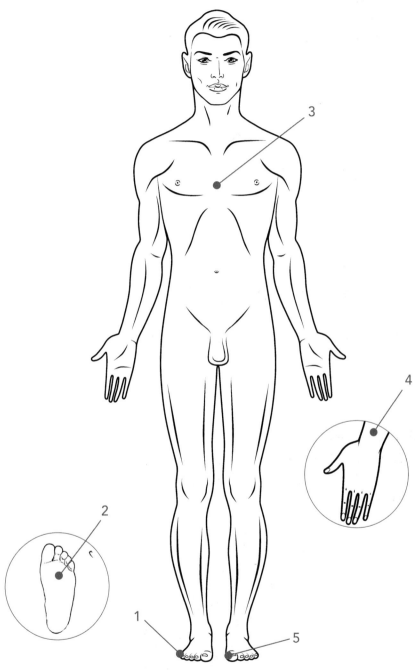

Circuit 3: Against Fear, Anxiety, and Panic

Circuit 4

Dealing with Obsessions

Most of us have experienced obsession to some degree: we have been in situations when everything seemed unimportant to us except that special thought that was occupying the entire space of our mind and would not go away even after a night's sleep.

That special thought generally concerns itself with love, business, weight issues, a break-up, or a disease, but whatever its cause, an obsessive thought always chases other mental faculties away and leaves no room for intuition or reason. We can't seem to focus any longer on our work or our life, and don't seem to mind if we seriously jeopardize our job and our relationships with our friends and family. We find that we have become unable to communicate and to listen to people. Basically, we just cut ourselves off from the world.

It is not uncommon for couples to split because of the absolute lack of communication arising from obsession: women find it particularly hard to live through a pregnancy all alone because their husbands are deep into their own problems.

Clearly the priority is to let go.

Point 1: Conception Vessel 4

(On the midline between the top of the pubis and the navel.)

This point is located on the center axis of the body, almost midway between the top of the pubic bone and the navel.

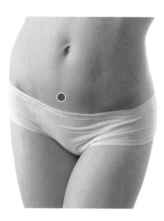

CV 4

Point 2: Governing Vessel 23

(From the anterior hairline follow the sagittal line of the skull back until a depression is felt at the anterior fontanel.)

This is the same as point 5 of circuit 2 against negativity; it is a slight depression situated on top of your cranium, some centimeters back from your hairline, right on the midline.

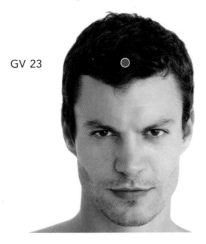

GV 23

Point 3: Large Intestine 4 (Right)

(Between the 1st and 2nd metacarpals of the right hand, on the radial aspect of the middle of the 2nd metacarpal bone, at the highest spot of the muscle when the thumb and index fingers are brought close together.)

This is the same as point 2 of circuit 2 against negativity. Separate your right thumb from your index finger, point 3 is right in the middle of the little hollow.

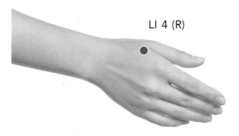

LI 4 (R)

Point 4: Lung 7 (Left)

(5 cm proximal to the most distal skin crease of the left wrist, proximal to the styloid of the radius in a depression between the bone and the tendons of brachioradialis and abductor pollicis longus.)

This is the same as point 4 of circuit 2 against negativity; it is located where we feel the pulse on the left wrist.

LU 7 (L)

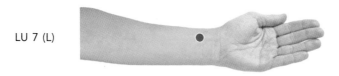

Point 5: Stomach 36 (Right)

(At the crest and to the external side of the right tibia just below the kneecap.)

Place the palm of your right hand on your right kneecap while keeping your right leg stretched. With your kneecap in the palm of your hand, notice the location of the end of your forefinger when you let it go toward the right of the most protuberant part of the major bone, the tibia; make sure you stay in contact with the outer edge of the bone. This is a tender spot. If it is not, don't break contact with the outer edge of the tibia, hold the pressure and feel around a little above and below until you detect sensitivity. Maintain the pressure for five seconds.

Alternatively, slowly follow the exterior edge of the crest of the tibia; at some point, you will feel a widening of this crest, near the knee joint; press firmly, pushing in the direction of the bone. The point is on the protuberance of the upper part of the muscle. You can't miss it.

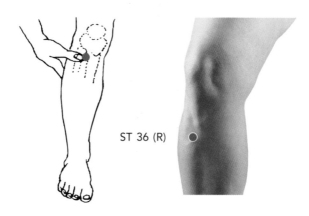

ST 36 (R)

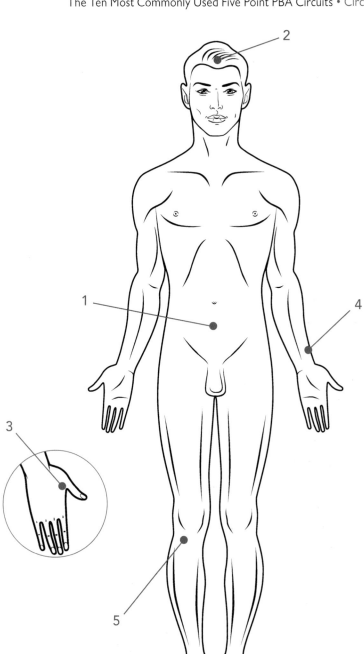

Circuit 4: Dealing with Obsessions

Circuit 5
_____

Against Hyper-Emotionality

This very important circuit is a much-used one. It helps with the management of our emotional fragility. When we find that we have become hypersensitive and that a very insignificant incident triggers our tears, then it may be the right moment to use circuit 5.

Or we can use this circuit when we realize that we are creating embarrassing situations through inappropriate highly emotional behavior (such as weeping uncontrollably and profusely at the happy ending of a movie, or when reminiscing about good times with friends). This category of incidents may not weigh very seriously in the balance of our lives, but they may make us feel exceedingly self-conscious and perhaps a little ridiculous; we may start being very apprehensive of a possible emotional outburst when going out for a movie night.

This circuit helps in the management of destabilizing situations as well. For example, my assistant felt very unwell one day after having been in contact with a highly negative person; she felt profoundly anxious and off-balance. I recommended that she do circuit 5, and sure enough, she recovered within five minutes and could go back to work.

Doing this circuit as soon as something unpleasant occurs helps to prevent the situation from taking unwanted proportions. It enables us to immediately recover our resourcefulness and potential to manage stress; we become able to tap into our courage in order to take the appropriate action. In other words, we can do whatever is necessary to deal with the situation and remain stable at the same time.

Point 1: Pericardium 6 (Right)

(On the anterior forearm, 5 cm proximal to the transverse wrist crease, between the tendons of palmaris longus and flexor carpi radialis.)

Place the first three fingers of the left hand on the inside of the wrist of your right hand. Slightly flex your right hand: you will distinctly feel two tendons. Press right between them, about five centimeters from the wrist crease.

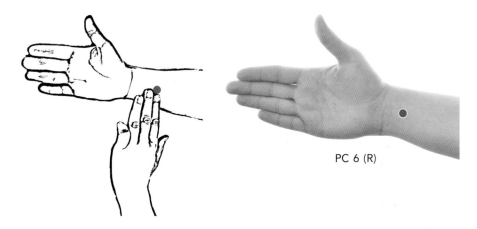

PC 6 (R)

Point 2: Triple Heater 5 (Left)

(On the left wrist, 5 cm proximal to the dorsal wrist crease between the radius and ulna, close to the radial bone.)

This is the same as point 4 of circuit 3 against fear, anxiety, and panic. Place your left hand upon your right shoulder; firmly hold your shoulder: now, place your left arm close against your chest. This enables you to uncross the two bones of your left forearm. Now, with the first three fingers of your right hand, press right between the two bones (about five centimeters from the base of your wrist). This is about where a watch usually rests.

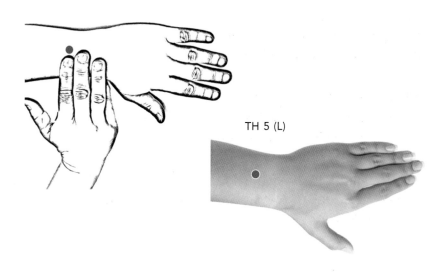

TH 5 (L)

Point 3: Small Intestine 8 (Right)

(With the elbow flexed, between the tip of the olecranon of the ulna and the tip of the medial epicondyle of the humerus.)

Flex your right elbow to make a right angle; you will feel a groove on the internal face (the one that faces your body), between the lower end of the humerus, the bone in your upper arm and the upper pointed end of the ulna (one of the two bones of your forearm). This is the spot to press. You may feel the cubital nerve roll under your fingers in an unpleasant way. In case of difficulty, don't hesitate to open and close your elbow a few times while keeping your thumb in the groove until you feel the right spot.

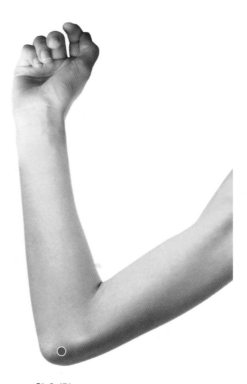

SI 8 (R)

Point 4: Lung 2 (Right)

(Inferior to the lateral extremity of the clavicle in a deep depression formed by the delto-pectoral triangle.)

To find this point, first follow the trajectory of your right collarbone, toward your shoulder. There, you'll find a little depression, which can be relatively deep; this depression is situated under the external part of the collarbone, just within the big round mass that corresponds to the curve of the shoulder. Press firmly to awaken the sensitivity that corresponds to the point you are seeking.

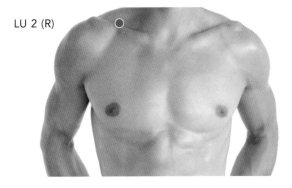

LU 2 (R)

Point 5: Governing Vessel 23

(From the anterior hairline follow the sagittal line of the skull back until a depression is felt at the anterior fontanel.)

This is the same as point 5 of circuit 2 against negativity and point 2 of circuit 4 against obsession; it is a slight depression situated on top of your cranium, some centimeters back from your hairline, right on the midline.

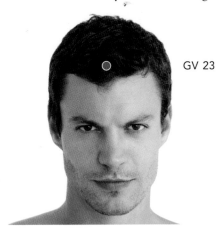

GV 23

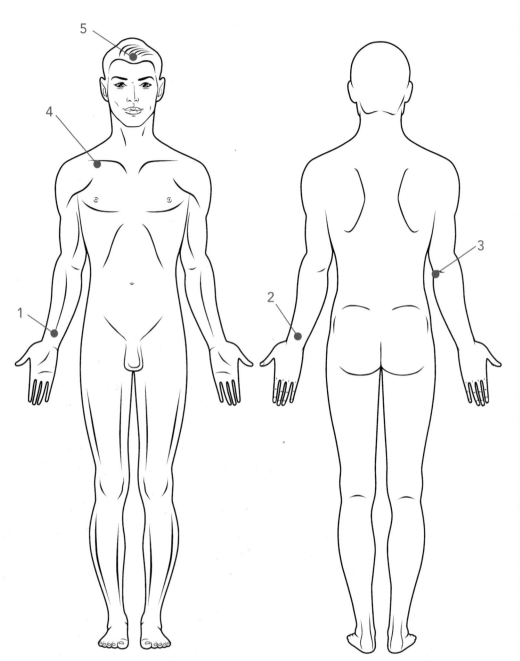

Circuit 5: Against Hyper-Emotionality

Removing Scars from Our Energetic System

Most of us have numerous scars on our energetic systems that have been produced by previous traumatic events. Any event that at some point has been experienced as traumatic has been encoded within us; because of the energetic nature of thought, serious incidents (or incidents perceived as serious) are connected with a significant release of energy that causes our "fuses" to "blow." The result is that our energetic system becomes abnormal.

This circuit is capable of clearing our scars and of resetting our system back to normal. The nature of the causal event that has been experienced as distressing does not really matter. In five point touch therapy the objective is not to pinpoint the origins of the issue; it is to "reset" the system and make it work again. It is like when the fuses blow in your house, you just want your lights and small appliances to work again; you are hardly interested in knowing whether a thunderstorm or a human error is responsible for the blackout.

If you are just beginning to work on yourself or on somebody else, it is of paramount importance that you apply this circuit. My long clinical observation has clearly shown that it is simply impossible for any of us to remain unscathed. This circuit should also be done each time you experience a traumatic emotional shock such as a breakup, a professional difficulty, or a loss.

This circuit eliminates the *energetic* consequences of what we have been through and have perceived as highly distressing; it will correct the imbalance of our energetic system and enable us to recover our potential for self-defense or survival. However, this circuit will not get rid of the *psychological* "scars" produced by a traumatic event or of its consequences on our current behavior. That particular work requires the expertise of other therapies such as behavioral therapy, sophrology, kinesiology, or five point touch therapy practiced by an accredited therapist who will use a specific technique that deals with the release of emotional blocks.

As for now and the purpose of this book, our objective is not the exploration of the causes of the incidents responsible for the imbalance of our energetic system. It is the management of temporarily upsetting emotions and the elimination of the energetic "scars" left by previous events by restoring the balance of our energetic system.

Point 1: Spleen 10 (Right)

(On the inner right thigh, five centimeters above the inferior extremity of the femur.)

On the inside of your right knee, feel the big bony protuberance at the lower end of your thigh bone. Proceed upward along your thigh for about five centimeters, then press deeply. You can't get it wrong, as this point is very sensitive most of the time.

If you are working on someone else, ask her to stretch her right leg and place your left hand on her right kneecap; the acupressure point will be right under your thumb.

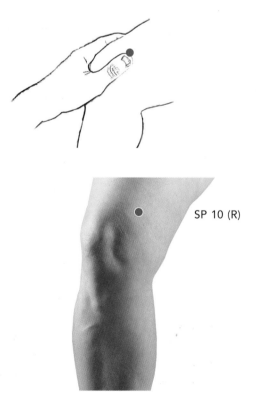

SP 10 (R)

Point 2: Gall Bladder 34 (Left)

(In a depression anterior and inferior to the head of the fibula.)

Feel the external part of your left leg, four to five centimeters below your knee, until you feel a bony protuberance that corresponds to the head of the fibula, the smaller bone of your lower leg. Feel a little depression a little underneath and slightly in front of this projection. Press there. As this is a tender spot, it is hard to miss.

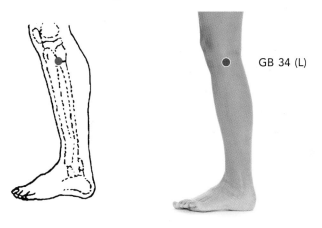

GB 34 (L)

Point 3: Liver 2 (Right)

(On the right foot, 2 cm proximal to the margin of the web of the 1st and 2nd toes.)

This point is located on the top of the right foot, just in the hollow between the first and second toes. If your pressure is strong enough, you will find that this point is extremely sensitive.

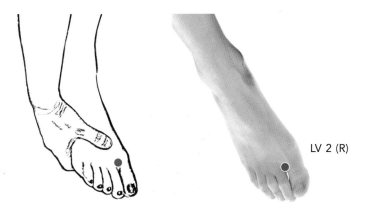

LV 2 (R)

Point 4: Urinary Bladder 62 (Right)

(Inferior to the lateral malleolus, in a depression posterior to the fibular tendons.)

On your right ankle (external side) search for the protuberance that forms the lower end of the fibula (smaller leg bone). Press just below this projection.

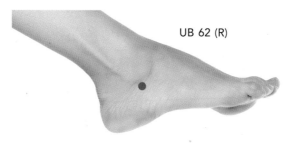

UB 62 (R)

Point 5: Spleen 6 (Left)

(On the internal side of the left ankle, 5 cm directly above the tip of the medial malleolus on the posterior border of the tibia.)

This is also point 1 in circuit 2 against negativity. It is situated on the inner side of the left ankle, about five centimeters above the prominence at the lower end of the tibia (larger lower leg bone).

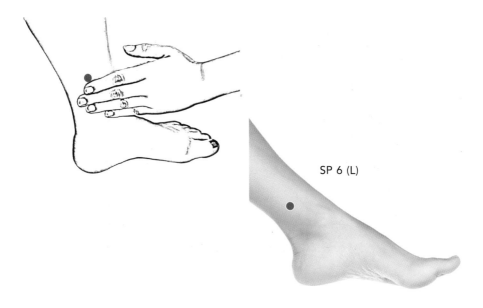

SP 6 (L)

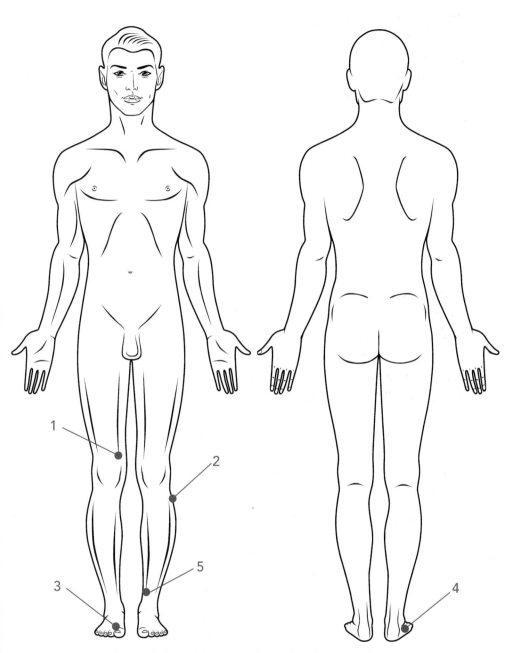

Circuit 6: Removing Scars from Our Energetic System

Circuit 7
___

Restoring the Fundamental Vibration

Once we are done with the elimination of negative energies, it's important that we positively "recharge" ourselves. Circuit 7 restores the balance of our seven energetic centers simultaneously; it allows the energy flow to regain fluidity and the energetic centers to vibrate in harmony.

This very important circuit is present in each of the protocols we'll study in chapter 4; each protocol must systematically end with it. Circuit 7 is the circuit that gives the final touch; it is indispensable and cannot be done without. Circuit 7 is also used specifically to deprogram those conditioning patterns that sabotage our life (to release emotional blocks).

Point 1: Pericardium 6 (Right)

(On the anterior forearm, 5 cm proximal to the transverse wrist crease, between the tendons of palmaris longus and flexor carpi radialis.)

Place the first three fingers of the left hand on the inside of the wrist of your right hand. Slightly flex your right hand: you will distinctly feel two tendons. Press right between them, about five centimeters from the wrist crease. This point is the same as point 1 in circuit 5 against hyper-emotionality.

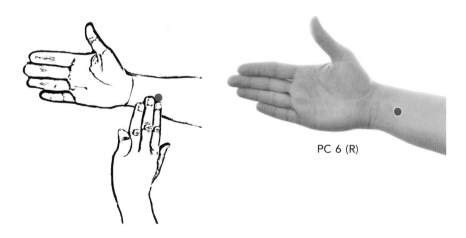

PC 6 (R)

Point 2: Urinary Bladder 2 (Left)

(On the medial end of the eyebrow, directly superior to the inner canthus of the eye, on the supraorbital notch.)

Start from your nose and feel the arch of your left eyebrow; with your thumb, follow the lower side of the arch; one or two centimeters from where your eyebrow begins, you will feel a little depression. This is point 2.

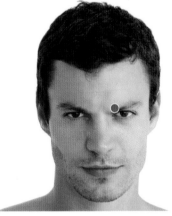

UB 2 (L)

Point 3: Special Point (Left Arm)

This point is not situated on a meridian. It is situated on the external side of your left forearm. First, press your left arm close to your chest. Six or seven centimeters from your elbow (this varies slightly from person to person) on the external side of your forearm, you will find a little depression that separates the two bones (this depression is visible in some cases); you may want to explore relatively deeply into the skin but this point is usually easy to locate.

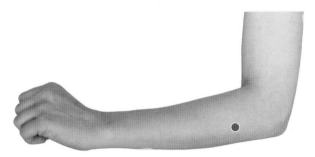

Point 4: Spleen 10 (Right)

(On the inner right thigh, five centimeters above the inferior extremity of the femur.)

On the inside of your right knee, feel the big bony protuberance at the lower end of your thigh bone. Proceed upward along your thigh for about five centimeters, then press deeply. You can't get it wrong, as this point is very sensitive most of the time. This is the same as point 1 in circuit 6 for removing the scars left by previous traumatic events.

On another person, you may want to try an alternative way to locate this point: with your left hand, enclose their right kneecap; the point lies right under your thumb.

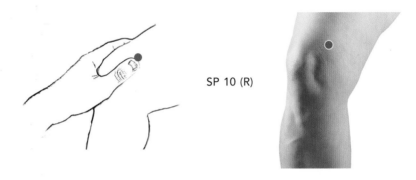

SP 10 (R)

Point 5: Gall Bladder 44 (Left)

(On the lateral side of the 4th left toe, 0.1 cm proximal to the margin of the nail.)

Just hold the fourth toe between the thumb and second finger and press firmly on the base of its nail.

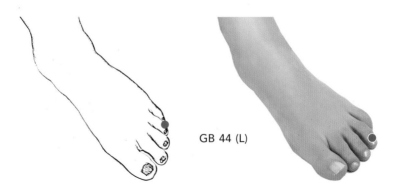

GB 44 (L)

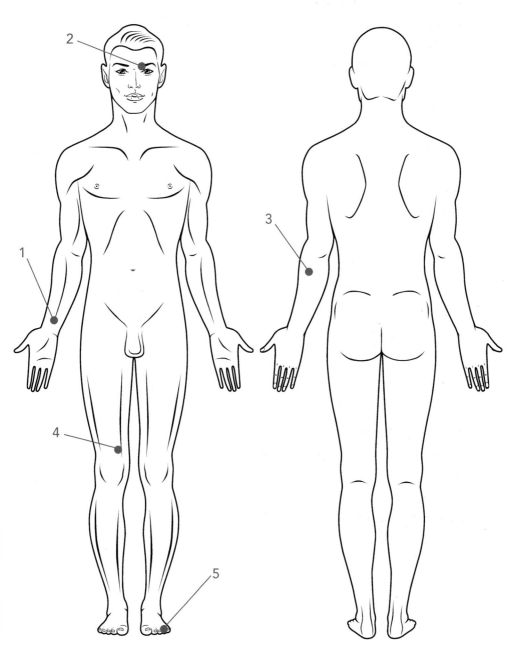

Circuit 7: Restoring the Fundamental Vibration

Circuit 8

Enhancing Expression

This circuit facilitates or enhances the faculties of expression, which often affect the success of a project. "Jitters" or extreme nervousness typically occur before an exam, a professional presentation, an entertainment show (if you are an actor), or a discussion with your bank manager. Jitters impede your faculties and cause failure of whatever you planned and needed to achieve. This circuit helps to stop the jitters.

Circuit 8 is also very useful if you feel that painful things have been bottled up for too long and that this lack of communication with your spouse, your boss, or your parents is becoming unbearable.

The zone of expression is obviously situated in the throat area, therefore expression issues have a good chance to cause somatic reactions in this region. Chronic throat issues are particularly customary in children. In adults, chronic expression issues commonly take the form of thyroid problems. This will be discussed when we present circuit 17, which more specifically deals with thyroid energies.

The following anecdote is amusing, as its pattern has become predictable: at the beginning of my workshops, participants are often a little shy and not very talkative. Inevitably though, once they have been taught circuit 8 and have experimented on themselves, the noise level intensifies significantly and everyone starts talking and bonding; this pattern occurs every time.

Point 1: Gall Bladder 34 (Left)
(In a depression anterior and inferior to the head of the fibula.)

The point is four to five centimeters below your left knee in a little depression just below and slightly in front of the projection at the top of the fibula. This is the same point as point 2 of circuit 6 for removing the scars from the energetic system.

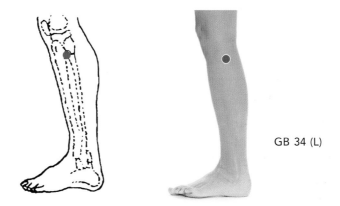

GB 34 (L)

Point 2: Spleen 6 (Right)

(On the internal side of the right ankle, 5 cm directly above the tip of the medial malleolus on the posterior border of the tibia.)

This is the symmetrical point of point 1 in circuit 2 against negativity and point 5 of circuit 6 against the energetic scars left by ancient trauma. It is situated on the inner side of the right ankle, about five centimeters above the prominence at the lower end of the tibia (larger lower leg bone). This point is often quite sensitive.

If you work on yourself place the little finger of your left hand on the bony projection: the point will be situated just under your index finger. Make sure you press upon the back edge of the tibia and *not* upon its front edge.

If you work on someone else, do as the sketch shows: put the little finger of your right hand on the bony projection; the point will be right under your index finger.

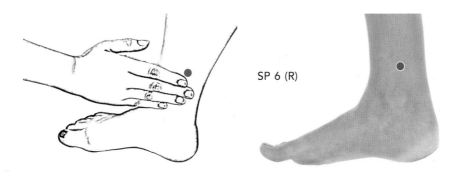

SP 6 (R)

Point 3: Triple Heater 5 (Left)

(On the left wrist, 5 cm proximal to the dorsal wrist crease between the radius and ulna, close to the radial bone.)

This point is situated on your left forearm at the place where a watch typically rests. This is the same as point 4 of circuit 3 against fear, anxiety, and panic and point 2 of circuit 5 against hyper-emotionality.

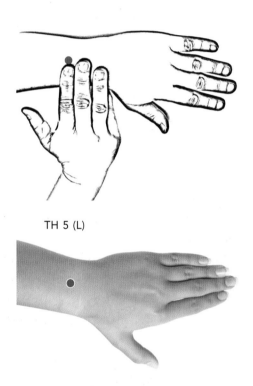

TH 5 (L)

Point 4: Stomach 36 (Right)

(At the crest and to the external side of the right tibia just below the kneecap.)

This is the same as point 5 of circuit 4 dealing with obsessions. Place the palm of your right hand on your right kneecap while keeping your right leg stretched. With your kneecap in the palm of your hand, notice the location of the end of your forefinger when you let it go toward the right of the most protuberant part of the major bone, the tibia; make sure you stay in contact with the outer edge of the bone. This is a tender spot. If it is not, don't break contact with the outer edge of the tibia, hold the pressure and feel around a little above and below until you detect sensitivity. Maintain the pressure for five seconds.

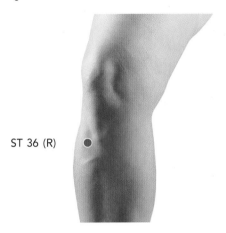

ST 36 (R)

Point 5: Urinary Bladder 2 (Left)

(On the medial end of the eyebrow, directly superior to the inner canthus of the eye, on the supraorbital notch.)

Start from your nose and feel the arch of your left eyebrow; with your thumb, follow the lower side of the arch; one or two centimeters from where your eyebrow begins, you will feel a little depression. This is the same as point 2 of circuit 7 for restoring the fundamental vibration.

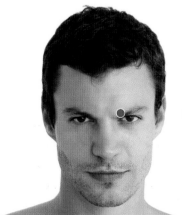

UB 2 (L)

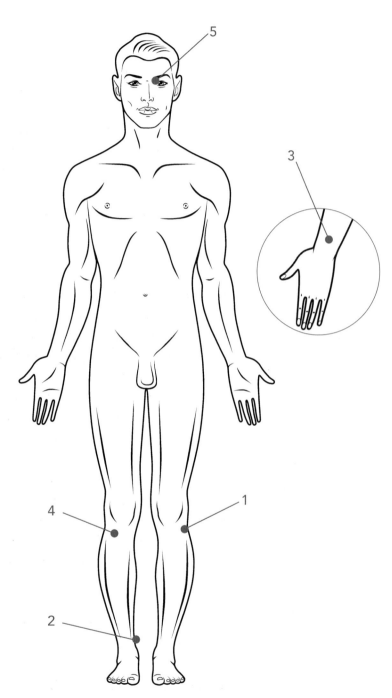

Circuit 8: Enhancing Expression

Restoring the Yin/Yang Balance

As mentioned in chapter 1, our body energies belong to two differentiated polarities: yin and yang. According to Chinese traditional knowledge, meridians are either yin or yang, yin being a more feminine polarity and yang a more masculine one. As a consequence, women should ideally be more yin and inversely, men should be more yang. If one polarity within us becomes more important than it should, our emotional and relational systems will be affected. Using circuit 9 to make sure that the balance is maintained is thus a good habit to have.

Circuit 9 is also used to correct weight issues, particularly when there is no endocrine or psychosomatic cause. The correction of the imbalance of yin and yang activates metabolism and allows weight to come down. Releasing the related emotional blocks can also really help. Weight gain is commonly a response to anxiety: our primitive brain is incapable of analyzing the real source of anxiety and automatically sends commands to the body to "stock up" on food (remember that one of the most primitive and primary human fears is starvation). Weight gain can also be a symbolic way to shield oneself from the world (when one lives in fear of being attacked), or it can be a result of an unconscious decision to make oneself sexually unattractive and unlikeable (once again for protection).

I consider this circuit as the "cherry on the cake": usually circuit 7 ends any procedure being used to clean up the energetic system (circuit 7 deals with the restoration of the fundamental vibration). If time allows it, the use of circuit 9 procures an added advantage; my patients always feel significantly more relaxed and balanced after it has been done.

Point 1: Spleen 4 (Right)

(On the medial side of the foot, in the depression distal and inferior to the base of the 1st metatarsal bone, at the junction of the light and dark skin.)

Follow the curve of the inner side of your right foot; you will feel a little depression on top of the curve. This depression corresponds to the base of the first metatarsal bone. Be careful, as this is a tender spot.

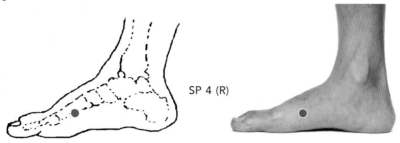

SP 4 (R)

Point 2: Spleen 10 (Left)

(On the inner left thigh, five centimeters above the inferior extremity of the femur.)

This point is symmetrical to the point above the right knee, which is point 1 of circuit 6 for removing scars of the energetic system and point 4 of circuit 7 used to restore the fundamental vibration. On the inside of your left knee, feel the big bony protuberance at the lower end of your thigh bone. Proceed upward along your thigh for about five centimeters, then press deeply. You can't get it wrong, as this point is very sensitive most of the time.

You may want to try an alternative way to locate this point: with your right hand, enclose the left kneecap; the point lies right under your thumb. This last technique is useful only when you work on another person.

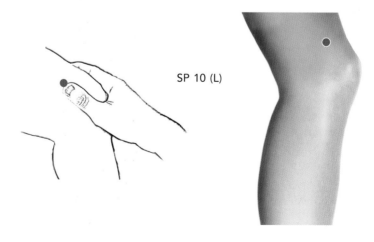

SP 10 (L)

Point 3: Large Intestine 4 (Right)

(Between the 1st and 2nd metacarpals of the right hand, on the radial aspect of the middle of the 2nd metacarpal bone, at the highest spot of the muscle when the thumb and index fingers are brought close together.)

This is the same point as point 2 of circuit 2 against negativity and point 3 of circuit 4 used to deal with obsessions. Separate your right thumb from your index finger, point 3 is right in the middle of the little hollow.

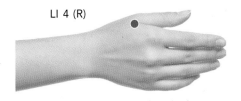

LI 4 (R)

Point 4: Stomach 36 (Right)

(At the crest and to the external side of the right tibia just below the kneecap.)

This is the same as point 5 of circuit 4 dealing with obsessions and point 4 of circuit 8 that enhances expression. Stretch your leg to locate it below the kneecap.

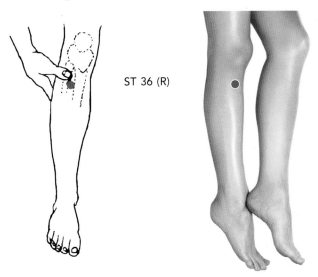

ST 36 (R)

Point 5: Urinary Bladder 67 (Right)

(Lateral aspect of the right little toe, 0.1 cm proximal to the corner of the nail.)

To locate this point, firmly hold your right little toe between the thumb and the second finger of your right hand; carefully place your thumb upon the last phalanx, just before the corner of the nail and press firmly. This is the same as point 1 of circuit 3 against fear.

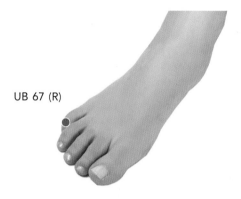

UB 67 (R)

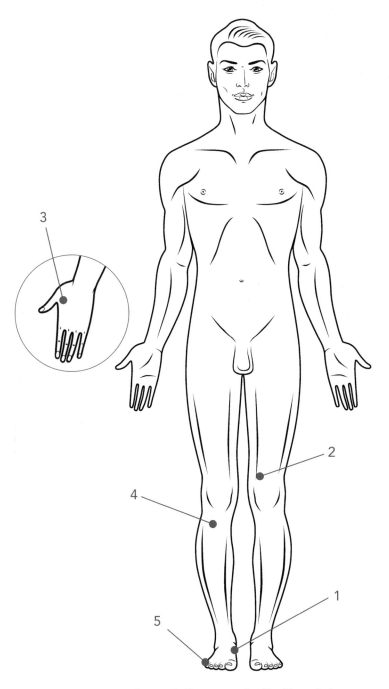

Circuit 9: Restoring the Yin/Yang Balance

Circuit 10

Against Suppressed Anger

Circuit 10 is the last circuit I added to the already existing set of circuits.

According to popular knowledge, anger is a bad adviser. From an energetic perspective, nothing is truer. Our energetic system responds to our emotions. Its integrity is maintained through positive thoughts; however, suppressed anger is so potent that it inhibits the action of the other previously introduced circuits as well as the action of the protocols given in chapter 4. This is how strong it is.

Suppressed anger may be pervasive: fury, suspicion, jealousy, even hatred are related problems to be taken into consideration as well. With it, negativity is total, leaving nothing unaffected; the face of the person, his language, his body language, and his general behavior express his state of mind. This particular situation is far worse than "simple" negativity (as treated by circuit 2) and has nothing to do with depression.

This is why, although circuit 10 is the last to be introduced, it has priority over all other circuits whenever you suspect your patient of being a victim of this peculiar energetic system. The case is not very common, but we must remember that the presence of suppressed anger is enough to make the action of the other circuits inoperative. Also, think about the possibility of suppressed anger whenever one of the protocols does not work as expected.

Point 1: Special Point (Abdomen)

(On the abdomen 1 cm above the umbilicus and 2 cm toward the patient's right.)

This special point is situated on your abdomen, about one centimeter above and two centimeters to the right of your navel.

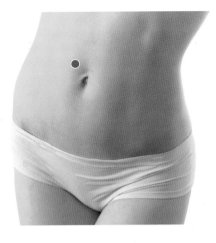

Point 2: Gall Bladder 34 (Left)

(In a depression anterior and inferior to the head of the fibula.)

The point is four to five centimeters below your left knee in a little depression just below and slightly in front of the projection at the top of the fibula. This is the same as point 2 of circuit 6 for removing the scars from the energetic system and point 1 of circuit 8 for enhancing expression.

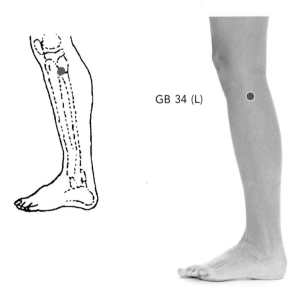

GB 34 (L)

Point 3: Spleen 6 (Left)

(On the internal side of the left ankle, 5 cm directly above the tip of the medial malleolus on the posterior border of the tibia.)

This point is the same as point 1 in circuit 2 against negativity. It is situated on the inner side of the left ankle, about five centimeters above the prominence at the lower end of the tibia (larger lower leg bone).

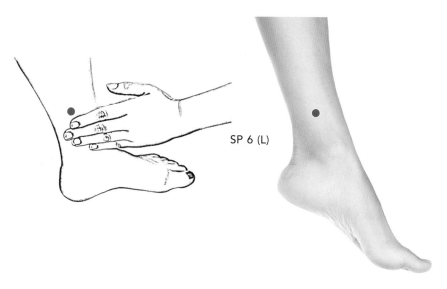

SP 6 (L)

Point 4: Large Intestine 4 (Right)

(Between the 1st and 2nd metacarpals of the right hand, on the radial aspect of the middle of the 2nd metacarpal bone, at the highest spot of the muscle when the thumb and index fingers are brought close together.)

We are quite familiar with this point by now; it is the same as point 2 of circuit 2 against negativity, point 3 of circuit 4 used to deal with obsessions, and point 3 of circuit 9 that restores the yin/yang balance.

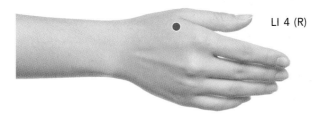

LI 4 (R)

Point 5: Special Point (Left Foot)

(Left foot, between the extensor tendons of the third and fourth toes, about 2 cm from their base.)

This point is on the back of the left foot, about two centimeters from the base of the toes, between the tendons of the third and fourth toes. This is symmetrical to point 3 of circuit 2 against negativity.

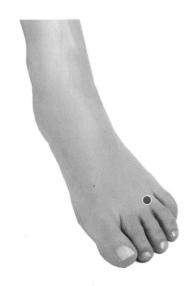

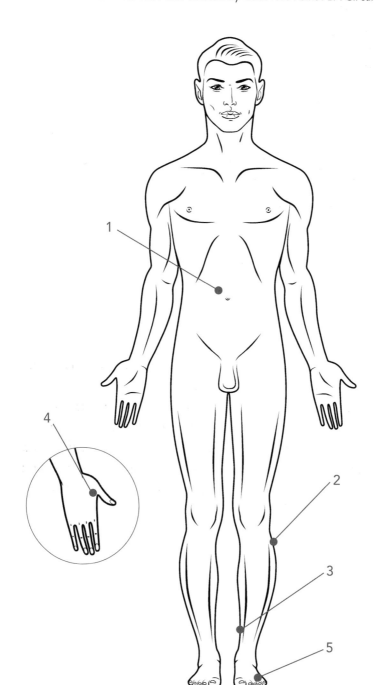

Circuit 10: Against Suppressed Anger

3
Twelve Additional Five Point PBA Circuits

The ten main circuits help us to manage the major part of the emotionally challenging situations we are bound to experience.

However, a certain number of less common situations may occur, such as a frustrating loss of creativity, and different cases of psychosomatic reactions (such as allergies, eczema, acne, bedwetting, colitis, and all sorts of conditions that are directly tied to our emotional state and sabotage our lives). PBA can help with those cases. Let us go into detail now.

Restoring the Energetic Coordination of the Brain

This circuit restores energetic coordination between the two hemispheres of the brain. Basically, let us just say here that the right brain is the intuitive one and that the left brain is the reasoning one. In order to work properly and ideally, our intuition should guide our reasoning, and reason should temper our intuition. An incorrect coordination can cause attention deficit and training difficulties. This has been scientifically demonstrated, and numerous techniques (kinesiology, eye movements) try to alleviate those connection problems.

This circuit proves to be very helpful particularly regarding young people. I have frequently worked with children affected by attention deficit disorder; these children found it hard or impossible to stay quiet for a minimum length of time and their memory was usually quite poor. Their parents were against the idea of specialized psychiatry despite the insistence of the teaching staff. I have used this specific circuit for almost two decades and I am in a position now to affirm its real efficacy in improving the situation of children who are affected by attention deficit disorder. Circuit 11 also helps with dyslexia, which in numerous cases has been demonstrated to be related to an incorrect energetic connection between the two hemispheres of the brain.

CASE STUDY
Attention Deficit

Eight-year-old Julien and his visibly very anxious mother came to consult me: week after week, Julien had been called to the principal's office. Invariably, he was reported to be constantly agitated, disturbing the whole class, and his constant daydreaming did not exactly help with the concentration he was supposed to have at school. In a word, little Julien could definitely not adapt to the rhythm of a mainstream class and was unable to focus on anything; his attention span was alarmingly short.

The same situation had been prevailing for years. At home, Julien could not remain collected for a minute, and if, by a miracle, lessons had been learned, they were forgotten the next day.

Working with a speech therapist and a specialist in graphology had given no results. The boy was labeled hyperactive and the drug Ritalin was recommended by his doctor. The mother refused the advice and came to see me without raising her hopes too high.

Before applying the classic Panic Protocol, I applied the five point circuit that restores the coordination between the two hemispheres of the brain. Then, I applied the circuit against fear because I had detected an underlying depression, which was not really a surprise as the boy was forever being scolded and considered an antisocial child.

Julien did get better rapidly and never needed a psychiatric treatment.

Point 1: Conception Vessel 24

(In the depression in the center of the mentolabial groove, inferior to the middle of the lower lip.)

This point is in the depression in the center of the groove below the lower lip.

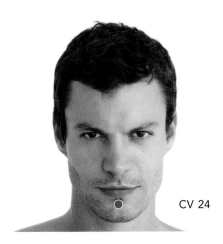

CV 24

Point 2: Spleen 14 (Right)

(Midway between the umbilicus and the superior part of the right hipbone.)

Picture an imaginary line between your navel and the top part of your right hipbone. Press right in the middle of this imaginary line.

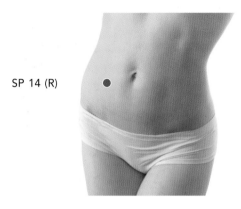

SP 14 (R)

Point 3: Triple Heater 5 (Left)

(On the left wrist, 5 cm proximal to the dorsal wrist crease between the radius and ulna, close to the radial bone.)

This point is situated on your left forearm at the place where a watch typically rests. We have met with this point a number of times now.

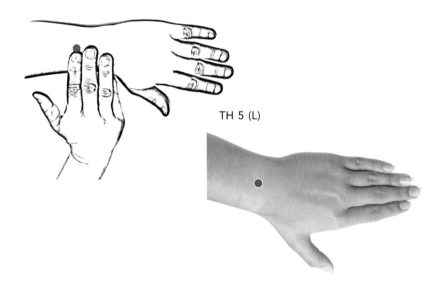

TH 5 (L)

Point 4: Stomach 36 (Right)

(At the crest and to the external side of the right tibia just below the kneecap.)

You are familiar with this point as well; it is the same as point 5 of circuit 4 dealing with obsessions and point 4 of circuit 8 that enhances expression. Stretch your leg to locate it below the kneecap.

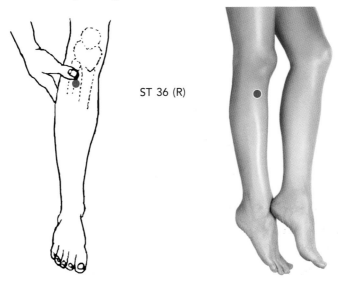

ST 36 (R)

Point 5: Special Point (Left Foot)

(Left foot, between the extensor tendons of the third and fourth toes, about 2 cm from their base.)

This point is on the back of the left foot, about two centimeters from the base of the toes, between the tendons of the third and fourth toes. It is the same as point 5 of circuit 10 against suppressed anger.

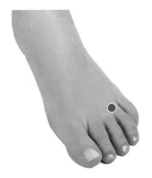

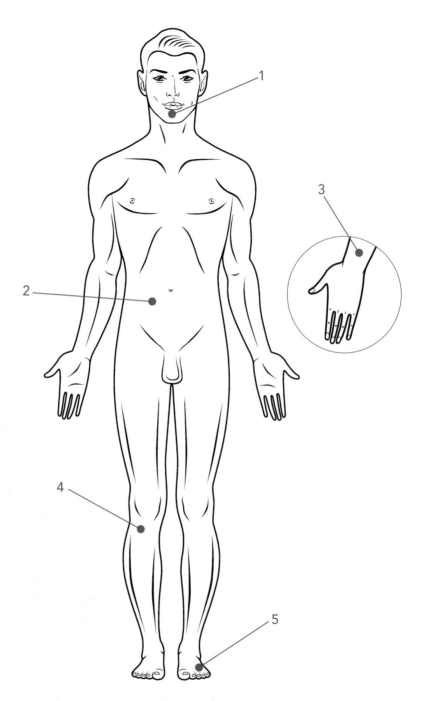

Circuit II: Restoring the Energetic Coordination of the Brain

Against Allergies Plus
Restoring the Ether Element

This is the first of three circuits that take care of skin problems.

Ayurvedic medicine, as well as other ancient traditions, speak of the existence of five elements: water, earth, fire, air, and ether (the Chinese replace the last two elements with wood and metal). These five elements symbolically correspond to each of the five senses. For example, fire is associated with eyesight and ether with touch. By extension, ether is associated with any skin problem such as allergies, eczema, or psoriasis. We may extrapolate and consider that even the respiratory allergies responsible for asthma are connected to a perturbation of the ether element.

The ether element is extremely sensitive to stress. It has become a well-known fact that eczema and particularly psoriasis are commonly linked to periods of strain or are reactivated by heavy pressure. In such cases, we have to concentrate first on the energies of panic (with that protocol) before taking care of the ether element and the related allergy problems. Therefore, this circuit should be preceded by either the Depression Protocol or Fear Protocol (depending on the case), and followed by the circuit against eczema. It will prove extremely useful in any case of skin allergy.

This circuit can also be tried in certain cases of asthma—the allergic kind, not the cardiac one—especially in children; anxiety-related, asthma often proves a psychosomatic disease that is reactivated by fresh causes for anxiety (as demonstrated by the considerable number of children suffering from an attack of asthma on the day of a school test they are apprehensive about). In working simultaneously on both anxiety and asthma, we have a chance to alleviate the attack.

Point 1: Lung 7 (Left)

(5 cm proximal to the most distal skin crease of the left wrist, proximal to the styloid of the radius in a depression between the bone and the tendons of brachioradialis and abductor pollicis longus.)

This is the same as point 4 of circuit 2 against negativity; it is located where we feel the pulse on the left wrist.

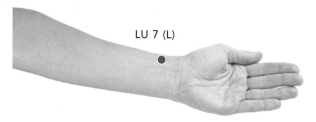

LU 7 (L)

Point 2: Triple Heater 5 (Right)

(On the right wrist, 5 cm proximal to the dorsal wrist crease between the radius and ulna, close to the radial bone.)

This point on the right forearm is symmetrical to point 4 of circuit 3 against fear, anxiety, and panic and point 2 of circuit 5 against hyper-emotionality.

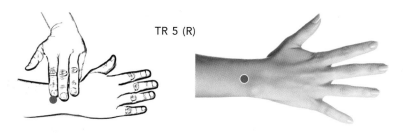

TR 5 (R)

Point 3: Liver 2 (Left)

(On the left foot, 2 cm proximal to the margin of the web of the 1st and 2nd toes.)

This point is located on the top of the left foot, just in the hollow between the first and second toes. It is symmetrical to point 3 of circuit 6 for removing scars from our energetic system.

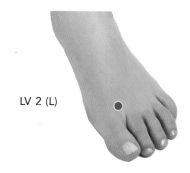

LV 2 (L)

Point 4: Triple Heater 10 (Left)

(With the elbow flexed, in a depression 1 cm superior to the olecranon.)

Flex your left elbow so as to form a right angle; you can distinctly feel three bony projections, which form the triangle (the inner and outer tips of the humerus and the tip of the ulna.) Press firmly right in the middle of this triangle.

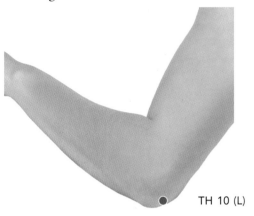

TH 10 (L)

Point 5: Stomach 36 (Right)

(At the crest and to the external side of the right tibia just below the kneecap.)

This point just below the knee should be well known also.

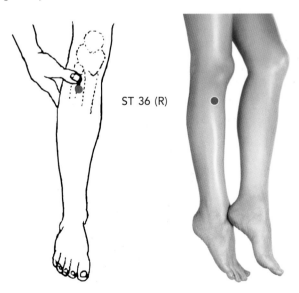

ST 36 (R)

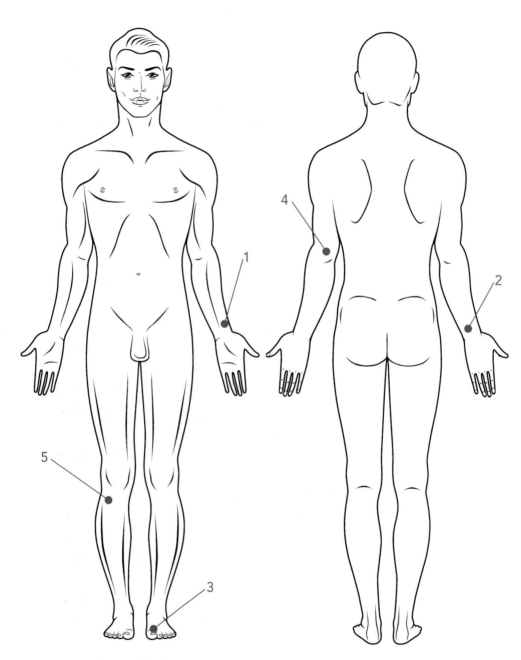

Circuit 12: Against Allergies Plus Restoring the Ether Element

Against Eczema

Eczema is a disabling disease, which is very painful to live with. The itching is terrible, particularly in case of extreme infection, and the esthetic prejudice is often experienced as unbearable. As it worsens during periods of pressure, it is easy to understand why, once there, eczema just does not go away. Its presence and the resulting discomfort generate more stress.

Some forms of eczema are evidently due to contact allergies: certain dyes or certain face creams may occasionally be responsible for skin problems. Clearly, the efficiency of the circuits decreases if contact with the particular products is not stopped.

Through my clinical experience over many years, I have observed that circuits 12 and 13 do bring a remarkable attenuation of certain forms of eczema. It is very important as well to do the circuits against fear, or even negativity, obsession, and sometimes depression, as all these emotional states are capable of producing an attack of eczema; the attack, in turn, is liable to create more anxiety. We will learn about the means to break this "vicious circle" in the next chapter, which is devoted to the impact of five point touch therapy on a certain number of psychosomatic diseases.

In the case of eczema it may also be good to eliminate dairy products (cheese, yogurt, and cream) from one's diet for at least three weeks. You could be in for a happy surprise. In the same way, think about the possibility of an allergy to lactose whenever a baby suffers from eczema. Talk to your doctor and together see whether an alternative baby food can be tried for a fortnight. (Soy milk could be considered an alternative.)

Note: Please don't hesitate to make use of the muscle testing described in chapter 2 in order to identify which products (such as cream, hair color, or food) you are allergic to.

CASE STUDY
Allergic Contact Eczema

Véronique was a forty-year-old beautician, who came to consult me in a state of intense dismay verging on depression.

Her hands were covered with an eczema that was painful and purulent. Not only was her condition aching but also her hands had become physically unsuitable for her job. Obviously, her eczema was caused by a contact of some sort; it was induced by an allergy to a product she was using regularly. Ideally, I would have suggested she stop using anything that could be irritating her skin, but then, her professional activity was at stake. Furthermore, the products she employed on a daily basis had all been lab tested without significant results.

But, like many beauticians, Véronique offered massages to her clients as a relaxation bonus. I asked her to bring me all the massage oils she was using; she had not mentioned those essential oils to the dermatologists because she thought them to be totally safe. Using muscle testing, I tested fifteen essential oils; three of those oils, including lavender, disturbed my patient on an energetic level.

I recommended that she stop using those three specific oils and I did the Panic and Depression Protocols, followed by the circuit that restores the ether element, as well, of course, as the one against eczema. Three weeks later, her eczema was gone, and she did not have to take any cortisone. (Cortisone is usually what is given to people suffering from serious allergies, though unfortunately, long-term side effects are not uncommon.)

In order to treat eczema, I recommend an application of circuit 13 several times during the day. The entire protocol for eczema (given in chapter 5 on page 160) should be done in the morning and possibly in the evening as well, but circuit 13 can be done any number of times during the day.

Point 1: Urinary Bladder 64 (Right)

(On the right foot, anterior and inferior to the lateral head of the 5th metatarsal.)

Point 1 is located on the external side of your right foot, in the little depression just in front of the upper end of the fifth metatarsal.

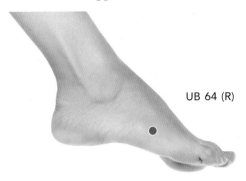

UB 64 (R)

Point 2: Governing Vessel 23

(From the anterior hairline follow the sagittal line of the skull back until a depression is felt at the anterior fontanel.)

We are familiar with this point. It is the same as point 5 of circuit 2 against negativity and point 2 of circuit 4 against obsession; it is a slight depression situated on top of your cranium, some centimeters back from your hairline, right on the midline.

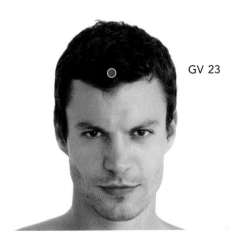

GV 23

Point 3: Lung 7 (Left)

(5 cm proximal to the most distal skin crease of the left wrist, proximal to the styloid of the radius in a depression between the bone and the tendons of brachioradialis and abductor pollicis longus.)

This is the same as point 4 of circuit 2 against negativity; it is located where we feel the pulse on the left wrist.

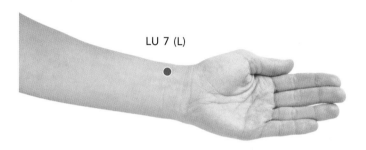

LU 7 (L)

Point 4: Triple Heater 5 (Right)

(On the right wrist, 5 cm proximal to the dorsal wrist crease between the radius and ulna, close to the radial bone.)

This point on the right forearm is symmetrical to point 4 of circuit 3 against fear, anxiety, and panic and point 2 of circuit 5 against hyper-emotionality.

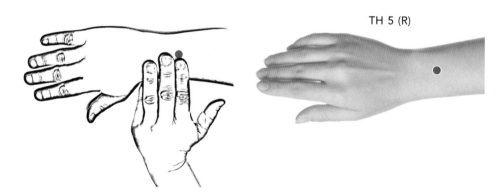

TH 5 (R)

Point 5: Pericardium 6 (Left)

(On the anterior forearm, 5 cm proximal to the transverse wrist crease, between the tendons of palmaris longus and flexor carpi radialis.)

Place the first three fingers of the right hand on the inside of the wrist of your left hand. Slightly flex your left hand: you will distinctly feel two tendons. Press right between them, about five centimeters from the wrist crease. This point is symmetrical to point 1 in circuit 5 against hyper-emotionality. The illustration below shows this point's relation to point 3 on the facing page.

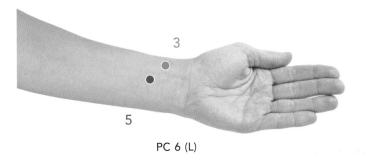

PC 6 (L)

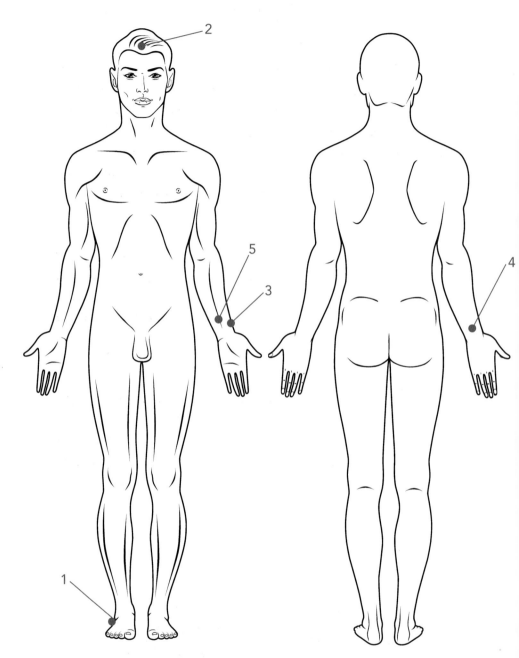

Circuit 13: Against Eczema

Circuit 14

Against Acne

This simple circuit has remarkable results. Teenagers are usually quite happy with it. Acne may be a real nuisance in their life and result in a sentiment of inferiority and hyper-sensitivity, which can highly disturb their future. Chemical treatments do exist of course, though they can occasionally prove aggressive and cause a dryness of the mucosa; sometimes, they can even be teratogenic. (*Teratogen* means any process or agent that causes the formation of developmental abnormalities in a fetus. Careful contraception is therefore required for a lengthy period of time after the use of any teratogenic treatment.)

My own children were taught this circuit during their teenage years and were quite satisfied with it. It can be applied by itself, without being preceded or followed by other circuits (if those are not needed of course.) It has to be done morning and evening, and, believe me, the adolescents to whom I taught it never forgot it!

Point 1: Spleen 6 (Left)
(On the internal side of the left ankle, 5 cm directly above the tip of the medial malleolus on the posterior border of the tibia.)

This point is the same as point 1 in circuit 2 against negativity. It is situated on the inner side of the left ankle, about five centimeters above the prominence at the lower end of the tibia (larger lower leg bone).

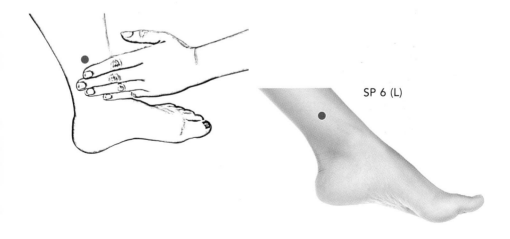

SP 6 (L)

Point 2: Urinary Bladder 2 (Right)

(On the medial end of the eyebrow, directly superior to the inner can-thus of the eye, on the supraorbital notch.)

Start from your nose and feel the arch of your right eyebrow; with your thumb, follow the lower side of the arch; one or two centimeters from where your eyebrow begins, you will feel a little depression. This is symmetrical to point 2 of circuit 7 for restoring the fundamental vibration.

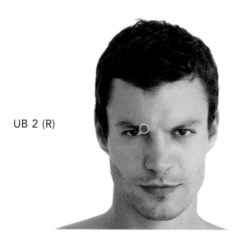

UB 2 (R)

Point 3: Large Intestine 4 (Left)

(Between the 1st and 2nd metacarpals of your left hand, on the radial aspect of the middle of the 2nd metacarpal bone, at the highest spot of the muscle when the thumb and index fingers are brought close together.)

Separate your left thumb from your index finger and exert pressure right in the middle. This is the same as point 4 in circuit 1 against depression.

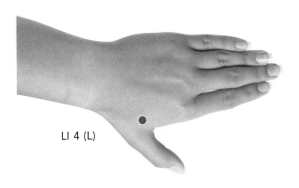

LI 4 (L)

Point 4: Stomach 7 (Right)

(In the depression at the lower border of the zygomatic arch, anterior to the condyloid process of the mandible.)

Place your right hand on your right cheek, and open your mouth. You can distinctly feel a little depression, which is formed between the lower and upper jawbones. This is where you must press.

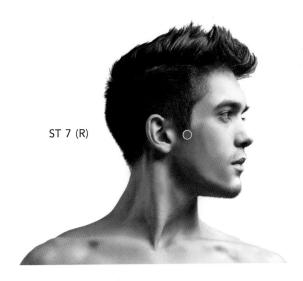

ST 7 (R)

Point 5: Gall Bladder 8 (Left)

(In a slight depression, 2 cm superior to the apex of the ear.)

Within the hairline, two finger-widths above and a little in front of the top of the left ear.

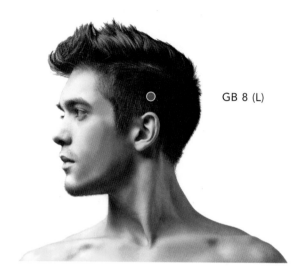

GB 8 (L)

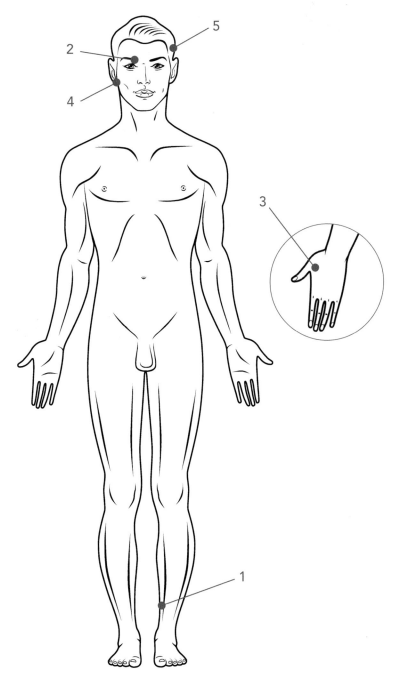

Circuit 14: Against Acne

Circuit 15

Energizing the Bladder

This circuit restores the balance of the energies of the bladder as well as its defense capacity; it can be used to fight against repetitive urinary infections such as cystitis.

Cystitis may often be related to infections, and also to psychological issues, and particularly to guilt; as guilt is an emotion that generates anxiety, it would be good to apply the appropriate circuits to clear those problems beforehand.

CASE STUDY

Cystitis and Feelings of Guilt

A young patient of mine used to suffer from cystitis every time she had intercourse.

Understandably, she grew extremely apprehensive and unable to relax before intercourse, and her relationship with her husband began to deteriorate. Years earlier, this young woman had been deserted by her first husband, and, although she had not been responsible for the separation, she could not help feeling guilty.

Though unconscious, this guilt was vivid; she had thus developed the idea of being adulterous each time she was in bed with her new partner. Deep in herself and without her conscious knowledge, she harbored this guilt and punished herself by putting her new relationship at risk.

This young woman's problem was solved thanks to the circuit that restores the energies of the bladder; she also realized that the source of her problem had been psychological.

Circuit 15 is also very useful to treat bedwetting in young children, as the problem is often behavioral. A child who wets his bed is an anxious child. If we keep in mind that urine has almost the same composition as the amniotic liquid, we can understand that wetting one's bed may be the way of the child's unconscious mind to recreate a safe environment that is a little similar to the womb.

If the time of pregnancy was an anxious time or if the birth was difficult, the child may be a little late in mastering a dry night; problems between her parents or moving from the first home may also be at the source of the issue.

Anxiety explains why many children who have already stopped wetting their bed suddenly lose control of their bladder all over again, once a baby sister or brother is born.

This attention-seeking behavior is clearly caused by two elements: on the one hand, the fear of abandonment and the fear of being deprived of their parents' love, and on the other hand, the unconscious will to remain babies themselves in order to counteract all the attention given to the newborn. In this case, this circuit has to be preceded by the Panic Protocol given in the next chapter.

Point 1: Urinary Bladder 64 (Left)

(On the left foot, anterior and inferior to the lateral head of the 5th metatarsal.)

Point 1 is located on the external side of your left foot, in the little depression just in front of the upper end of the fifth metatarsal. This point is symmetrical to point 1 of circuit 13 against eczema.

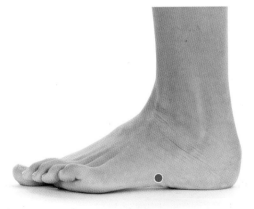

UB 64 (L)

Point 2: Kidney 3 (Right)

(On the right ankle in the depression between the medial malleolus and the Achilles tendon, level with the tip of the medial malleolus.)

This point is located on the inside of the right ankle, in the depression between the protruding lower end of the tibia and the Achilles tendon, level with the tip of the protrusion.

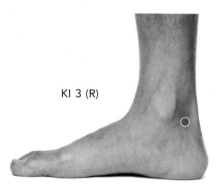

KI 3 (R)

Point 3: Small Intestine 8 (Left)

(With the elbow flexed, between the tip of the olecranon of the ulna and the tip of the medial epicondyle of the humerus.)

Flex your left elbow to make a right angle; you will feel a groove on the internal face (the one that faces your body), between the lower end of the humerus—the bone in your upper arm—and the upper pointed end of the ulna (one of the two bones of your forearm). This is the spot to press. You may feel the cubital nerve roll under your fingers in an unpleasant way. In case of difficulty, don't hesitate to open and close your elbow a few times while keeping your thumb in the groove until you feel the right spot. This point is symmetrical to point 3 of circuit 5 against hyper-emotionality.

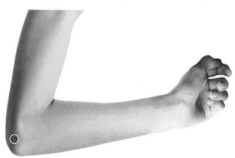

SI 8 (L)

Point 4: Stomach 36 (Right)
(At the crest and to the external side of the right tibia just below the kneecap.)

This should be a familiar point by now, just below the right kneecap.

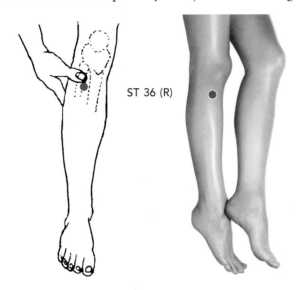

ST 36 (R)

Point 5: Spleen 6 (Left)
(On the internal side of the left ankle, 5 cm directly above the tip of the medial malleolus on the posterior border of the tibia.)

We are familiar with this point. It is situated on the inner side of the left ankle, about five centimeters above the prominence at the lower end of the tibia (larger lower leg bone).

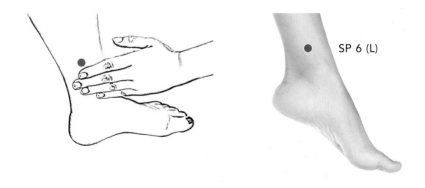

SP 6 (L)

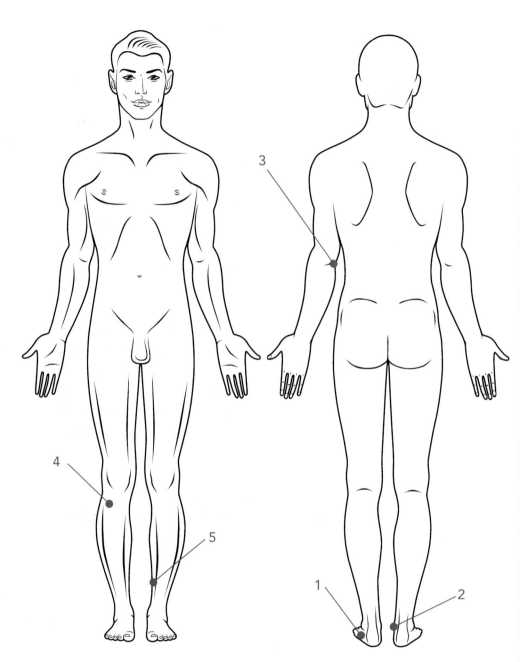

Circuit 15: Energizing the Bladder

Circuit 16

Energizing the Colon

The colon is *the* organ that symbolizes the psychosomatic reaction of anxiety at its best (or rather at its worst). It is usually extremely sensitive to fear and stress.

An anecdote concerning WW1 soldiers comes to my mind: a number of them were so terrified during the horrendous trench warfare that they could not control their sphincters at all. It is a well-known fact that people who suffer from colitis (those painful spasms of the large intestine) are people who suffer from high anxiety. (The intestine can be considered as the "third brain," the second one being the heart.)

Circuit 16 has also revealed itself very useful to alleviate the pains that result from the aftereffects of a parasitic (especially amoebic) colic or of painful chronic infections associated with the sigmoid colon (the S-shaped terminal part of the descending colon).

This circuit is also extremely helpful for treating colic in a baby, which is often linked, as previously said, to maternal anxiety that the baby felt while in the womb; colic may be related to a difficult birth as well. This type of colic is easily treated by applying circuit 16, preceded by the circuit 3 against fear (we'll see the detail of this in chapter 5, which provides a glossary of conditions and recommended protocols).

Point 1: Stomach 25 (Left)

(Level with the umbilicus, midway between it and the left side.)

Point 1 is level with the navel, about midway between it and your left side.

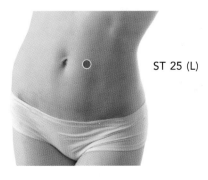

ST 25 (L)

Point 2: Liver 2 (Left)

(On the left foot, 2 cm proximal to the margin of the web of the 1st and 2nd toes.)

This point is located on the top of the left foot, just in the hollow between the first and second toes. It is the same as point 3 of circuit 12 against allergies.

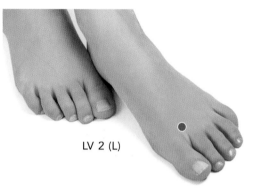

LV 2 (L)

Point 3: Large Intestine 4 (Right)

(Between the 1st and 2nd metacarpals of the right hand, on the radial aspect of the middle of the 2nd metacarpal bone, at the highest spot of the muscle when the thumb and index fingers are brought close together.)

We have seen this point a number of times before; it is located on the back of your right hand, between your thumb and your index finger.

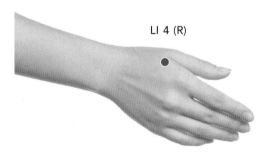

LI 4 (R)

Point 4: Gall Bladder 38 (Left)

(On the left ankle, about 8 cm above the tip of the lateral malleolus, on the anterior border of the fibula.)

Point 4 is located on the outside of your lower leg, about four finger-widths above the protruding end of the fibula.

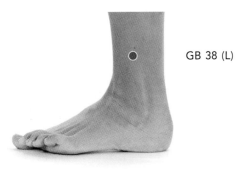

GB 38 (L)

Point 5: Spleen 6 (Right)

(On the internal side of the right ankle, 5 cm directly above the tip of the medial malleolus on the posterior border of the tibia.)

We should be very familiar with this point now. It is situated on the inner side of the right ankle, about five centimeters above the prominence at the lower end of the tibia (larger lower leg bone).

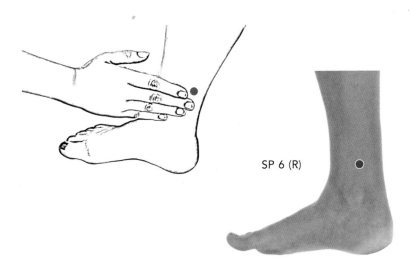

SP 6 (R)

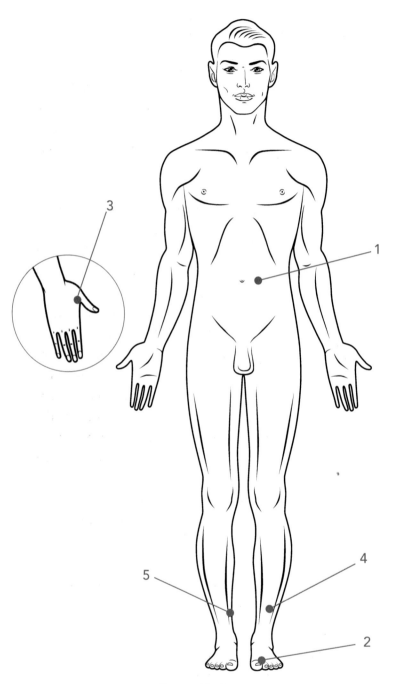

Circuit 16: Energizing the Colon

Circuit 17

Restoring Thyroid Function

Our thyroid gland is extremely fragile, so its most insignificant defect disturbs us. Its role in our metabolism is critical: we find ourselves all swollen when it does not function adequately, and we lose weight when it works in excess. It also plays a role in our character and way of being: if it does not work sufficiently, we feel listless and tired; in the opposite case, we are nervous and constantly agitated.

Stress and unexpressed feelings are responsible for the disturbance of the thyroid gland. The necessity for healthy verbal expression seems therefore all the more obvious. It is generally believed that verbal expression helps clear the destructive emotions that transform into diseases if they are left unexpressed. Many illnesses are responses to psychological strain. Researchers, particularly in the United States, have even concluded from their observations that people who keep diaries tended to be twice less liable to develop cancer than those who did not.

This is the reason why Jacques Salomé, famous French psychologist and psychotherapist, recommends the creation of "symbol-objects": these symbolic objects are used to represent a person with whom meaningful communication has been impossible in the past. Expressing the things that matter to us, even to an object, somehow tricks our brain, which works in a symbolic way and observes no difference between an imagined situation and a real one.

As we are dealing with energies, this technique is a really effective way to get rid of anger, anxiety, or aggressiveness. This helps to protect our organs; our thyroid especially remains safe.

CASE STUDY
The Use of Symbolic Objects

A relatively aged patient of mine had a serious issue with her eldest son; however, she did not feel like making matters worse, so she decided to say nothing about how she felt. Unsurprisingly, this unsolved situation soon got the better of her health and she started to lose excessive weight and spiral down toward depression.

I suggested that she make a symbolic object and so she did: she found an old wire owl in a drawer, put it on the kitchen table, and each time she walked in, she vehemently addressed the owl: "Why did you do that to your old mother? Don't you have any respect at all?" and so forth.

Amazing as this may sound, she completely recovered; she called me two weeks later to tell me how good and liberated she felt. After a few months, she consulted me again and confirmed that all was well with her son who was soon coming for a holiday to her place. I asked about the owl, to which she answered with humor: "I came to hate it so much that I got rid of it."

I smiled, because I knew that getting rid of the owl meant getting rid of all those destructive emotions she had somehow transferred to the object. Understandably, the owl then made her uncomfortable.

This anecdote speaks for the efficacy of the symbolic object; the whole idea seems a little far-fetched, but from an energetic perspective, it is an extraordinary tool. In case of issues with different persons, different symbolic objects have to be used; otherwise our brain will be confused and won't be tricked. This kind of symbolic object is far different from a confidant, or those favorite toys of our childhood to which we told our little secrets; its function is to represent a person with whom communication has been impossible.

To come back to the thyroid, circuit 17 won't restore a thyroid that is already affected by cysts and dystrophies; but in cases of slight malfunctioning it can restore things to normal and it is worth trying for some days before opting for a hormonal treatment. Or, in case of a more serious situation, it could in the long run help diminish the doses of drugs.

However, the use of this circuit should be mostly preventive: if you are aware of not expressing your true feelings and realize at the same time that you are losing weight and are very nervous (or, conversely, if you feel very tired and are putting on weight), then it's a good idea to do it systematically; remember that this circuit restores the balance of energies; before applying circuit 17, apply circuit 3 against fear and circuit 8 for encouraging expression.

Point 1: Lung 9 (Left)

(At the wrist crease on the radial side of the radial artery.)

This point is on the left wrist crease.

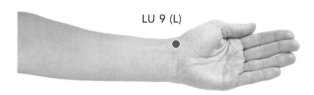

LU 9 (L)

Point 2: Special Point (Right Arm)

This point is not situated on a meridian. It is situated on the external side of your right forearm. First, press your right arm close to your chest. Six or seven centimeters from your elbow (this varies slightly from person to person) on the external side of your forearm, you will find a little depression that separates the two bones (this depression is visible in some cases); you may want to explore relatively deeply into the skin but this point is usually easy to locate. It is symmetrical to point 3 of circuit 7 for restoring the fundamental vibration.

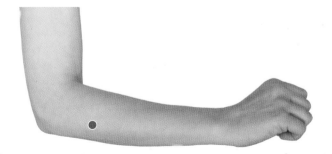

Point 3: Heart 9 (Left)

(On the radial side of the left little finger, 0.1 cm proximal to the corner of the nail.)

This point is located near the end of the little finger of the left hand, just at the lower corner of the nail on the side nearest the fourth finger.

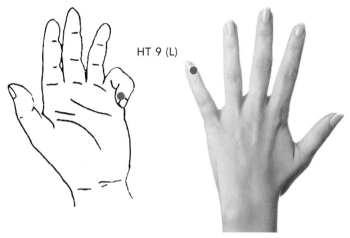

HT 9 (L)

Point 4: Stomach 41 (Left)

(On the ankle, level with the lateral malleolus, in the depression between the tendons of the extensor digitorum longus and halluces longus muscles.)

This point is located in the center of the top of the left ankle, in the depression between the two tendons.

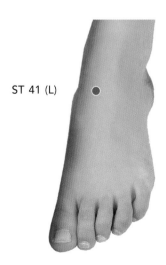

ST 41 (L)

Point 5: Spleen 6 (Right)

(On the internal side of the right ankle, 5 cm directly above the tip of the medial malleolus on the posterior border of the tibia.)

We should be very familiar with this point now. It is situated on the inner side of the right ankle, about five centimeters above the prominence at the lower end of the tibia (larger lower leg bone).

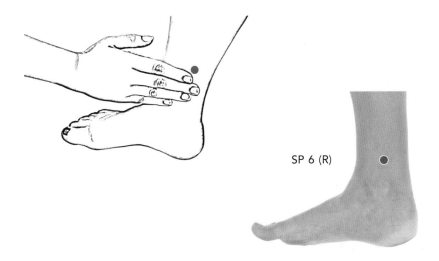

SP 6 (R)

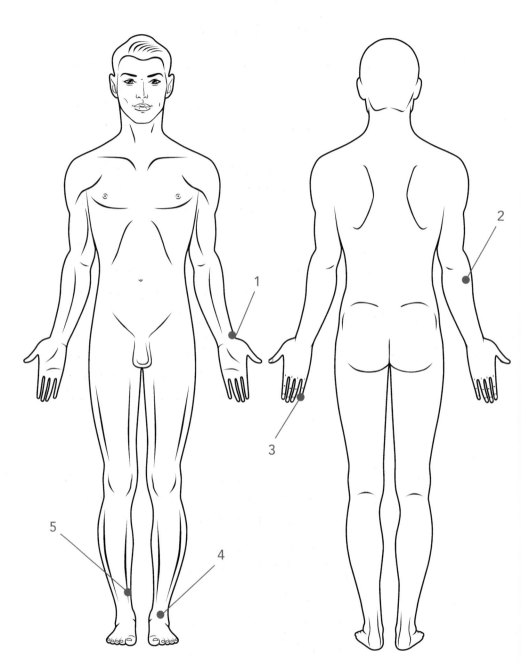

Circuit 17: Restoring Thyroid Function

Circuit 18

Stimulating Creativity

This is a major circuit for those who want to awaken or stimulate their creativity, but keep in mind that it has nothing to do with motivation. We know that the lack of motivation is a sign of depression. However, it's quite possible to lack a much-needed inspiration and at the same time feel highly motivated.

This circuit could be useful to a journalist, who has a deadline and finds it impossible to write her story; a painter, a writer, a composer—any person whose work requires inspiration or imagination—will find circuit 18 quite helpful.

In fact, the circumstances when we find ourselves in dire need of creativity are endless. There are many times when our intuition eludes us when we do need it in order to create whatever it is we wish to create. I for one have made use of circuit 18 whenever I felt I required it.

I had the opportunity to help a dear friend of mine, a painter who, despite being very gifted, had found himself "blocked" and unable to paint anymore; a few days after I worked on him, he started to paint again with a new-found inspiration, and two years later, his first exhibition in a long time was a success.

Point 1: Spleen 21 (Right)

(On the right side, on the mid-axillary line in the 6th intercostal space.)

Along the right side of the chest, in the space below the sixth rib. This point is easy enough to locate, as its sensitivity is rather high.

SP 21 (R)

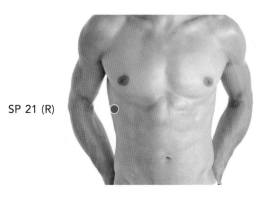

Point 2: Conception Vessel 4

(On the midline between the top of the pubis and the navel.)

This point is located on the center axis of the body, almost midway between the top of the pubic bone and the navel. This point is the same as point 1 of circuit 4 for dealing with obsessions.

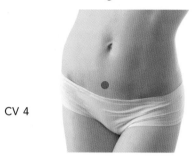

CV 4

Point 3: Kidney 3 (Left)

(On the left ankle in the depression between the medial malleolus and the Achilles tendon, level with the tip of the medial malleolus.)

This point is located on the inside of the left ankle, in the depression between the protruding lower end of the tibia and the Achilles tendon, level with the tip of the protrusion. This point is symmetrical to point 2 of circuit 15 for energizing the bladder.

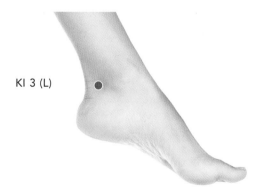

KI 3 (L)

Point 4: Lung 7 (Right)

(5 cm proximal to the most distal skin crease of the right wrist, proximal to the styloid of the radius in a depression between the bone and the tendons of brachioradialis and abductor pollicis longus.)

This is where your doctor usually feels your pulse. It is the same as point 3 of circuit 1 against depression.

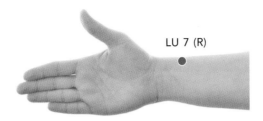

LU 7 (R)

Point 5: Stomach 36 (Left)

(At the crest and to the external side of the left tibia just below the kneecap.)

This is symmetrical to point 5 of circuit 4 for dealing with obsessions, point 4 of circuit 8 for enhancing expression, and others. Place the palm of your left hand on your left kneecap while keeping your left leg stretched. With your kneecap in the palm of your hand, notice the location of the end of your forefinger when you let it go toward the left of the most protuberant part of the major bone, the tibia; make sure you stay in contact with the outer edge of the bone. This is a tender spot. If it is not, don't break contact with the outer edge of the tibia, hold the pressure and feel around a little above and below until you detect sensitivity. Maintain the pressure for five seconds.

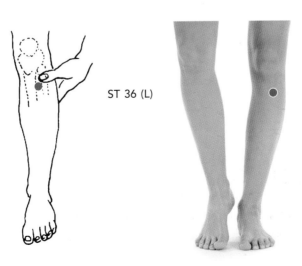

ST 36 (L)

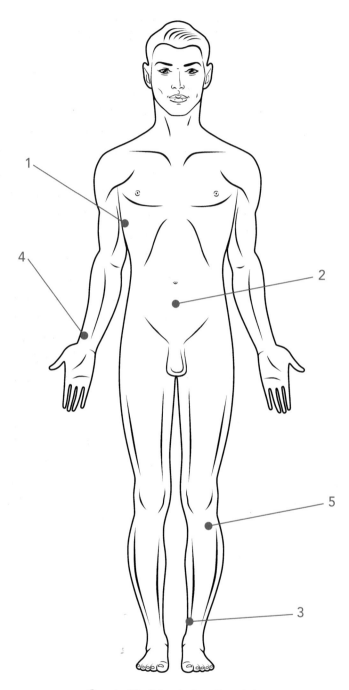

Circuit 18: Stimulating Creativity

Circuit 19

Energizing the Sacral Plexus

The sacral plexus corresponds to what is usually called "the root chakra." It has a crucial importance in psychosomatic matters, as it is the "power outlet" that feeds the uterus, the prostate, and the lumbar vertebrae, as well as the genital organs. The sacral plexus symbolizes determination, action, and safe and stable roots. It anchors us into our physical lives and helps us to stay grounded. Any type of situation that disrupts the three functions of tenacity, action, and secure structure or stable roots is liable to produce a dysfunction or even a disease that will affect the organs that depend on the sacral plexus.

A problem of "uprooting" may occur when we lose our sense of inner security and our usual references or bearings (such as can happen with a change of house or country, or a change in our way of life, such as a divorce or the loss of a job). If we are constantly bullied by our boss or endlessly frustrated in the choices we'd like to make, when we are submerged by the load of our responsibilities and can't find personal space, that may pave the way for future lumbago, sciatica, or possibly uterus or prostate issues.

Other related conditions are linked to the loss of energy at the level of the sacral plexus and are psychosomatic par excellence: diverse sexual problems, such as impotence, premature ejaculation, or frigidity, which simultaneously concern the first and second energy centers.

Preventive care of our sacral plexus is definitely a good idea, especially if we experience a situation in which we feel insecure.

Point 1: Special Point (Left Foot)

(Left foot, between the extensor tendons of the third and fourth toes, about 2 cm from their base.)

This point is on the back of the left foot, about two centimeters from the base of the toes, between the tendons of the third and fourth toes. It is the same as point 5 of circuit 10 against suppressed anger and point 5 of circuit 11 for restoring the energetic connection of the hemispheres of the brain.

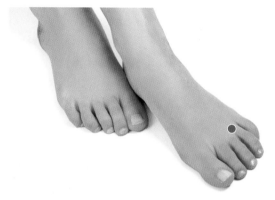

Point 2: Stomach 36 (Right)

(At the crest and to the external side of the right tibia just below the kneecap.)

This should be a familiar point by now, just below the right kneecap.

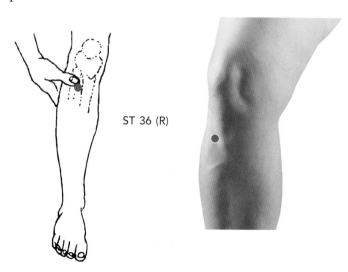

ST 36 (R)

Point 3: Kidney 6 (Right)

(On the inner right ankle, 1 cm inferior to the tip of the medial malleolus, in a depression formed by two ligamentous bundles.)

This point is on the inner right ankle just below the lower tip of the protrusion at the lower end of the tibia.

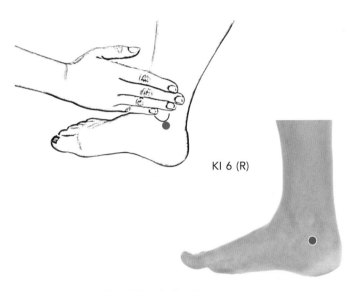

KI 6 (R)

Point 4: Urinary Bladder 2 (Left)

(On the medial end of the eyebrow, directly superior to the inner canthus of the eye, on the supraorbital notch.)

This point on the left eyebrow is the same as point 2 of circuit 7 for restoring the fundamental vibration.

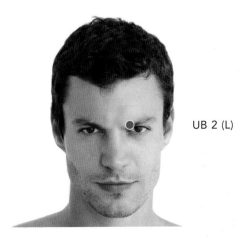

UB 2 (L)

Point 5: Spleen 6 (Right)

(On the internal side of the right ankle, 5 cm directly above the tip of the medial malleolus on the posterior border of the tibia.)

We should be very familiar with this point now. It is situated on the inner side of the right ankle, about five centimeters above the prominence at the lower end of the tibia (larger lower leg bone). The illustration below shows this point's relation to point 3 on the previous page.

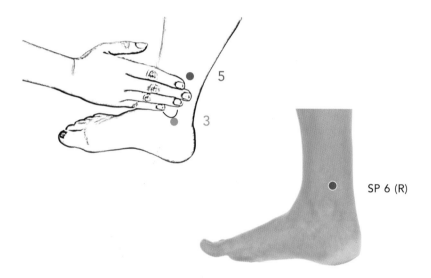

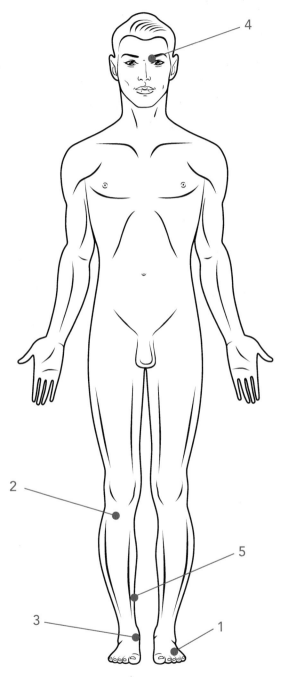

Circuit 19: Energizing the Sacral Plexus

Energizing the Solar Plexus

The well-known feeling of having a weight on one's stomach is the way that our solar plexus warns us that something is wrong with us; at times, the anxiety level is so high that breathing becomes hard. The solar plexus harbors our deep sense of self and our freedom of choice.

The solar plexus corresponds to our third energetic center; it is responsible for "feeding" the whole upper part of our digestive sphere (the liver, the stomach, the pancreas, and the gallbladder). Its dysfunction results in a certain number of psychosomatic diseases, especially where these organs are concerned.

Like the sacral plexus and the thyroid, the solar plexus is hypersensitive to anxiety. However, the sacral plexus reacts to actual events, events that happen in physical reality and active life, whereas the thyroid is affected by expression issues and unspoken feelings. Things are different again with the solar plexus, which is responsive to a form of anxiety that has no known source: you just feel anguished, as though this emotion were a second nature; angst becomes chronic as though it is almost part of your character.

We know that worried people are susceptible to stomach ulcers and, in the long run, may develop gallbladder stones. In medical literature, there are even cases of stress diabetes: diabetes just emerges after a breakup or a failed exam; the pancreas, deprived of energy, has just stopped working. The disturbance of the solar plexus is also responsible for numerous problems of metabolism or even obesity, due to the dysfunction of the whole digestive system that has been generated.

It is therefore of paramount importance to take care of the harmonious working of your solar plexus, especially if you are subject to anxiety. This circuit is important as well when, in spite of the daily application of the Panic Protocol (described in the next chapter), sensitivity is still felt in the pit of the stomach or underneath the right rib, in the area of the gallbladder.

Point 1: Special Point (Upper Left Abdomen)

(Beneath the last left rib, on the mid-axillary axis.)

This point is found beneath the last left rib, on the axis that connects the left armpit with the top of the left hip.

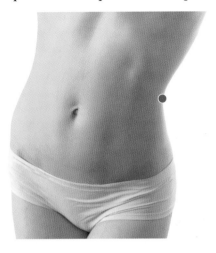

Point 2: Spleen 6 (Left)

(On the internal side of the left ankle, 5 cm directly above the tip of the medial malleolus on the posterior border of the tibia.)

This is the same as point 1 in circuit 2 against negativity. It is situated on the inner side of the left ankle, about five centimeters above the prominence at the lower end of the tibia (larger lower leg bone).

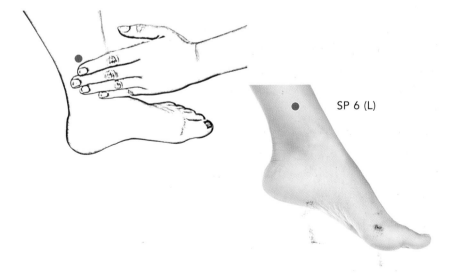

SP 6 (L)

Point 3: Urinary Bladder 2 (Left)

(On the medial end of the eyebrow, directly superior to the inner canthus of the eye, on the supraorbital notch.)

This point on the left eyebrow is the same as point 2 of circuit 7 for restoring the fundamental vibration.

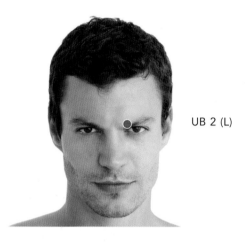

UB 2 (L)

Point 4: Stomach 36 (Right)

(At the crest and to the external side of the right tibia just below the kneecap.)

This should be a familiar point by now, just below the right kneecap.

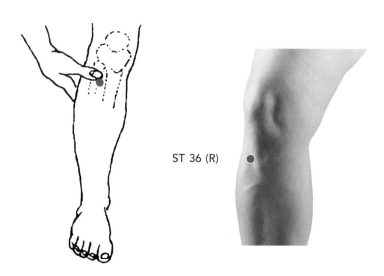

ST 36 (R)

Point 5: Triple Heater 5 (Right)

(On the right wrist, 5 cm proximal to the dorsal wrist crease between the radius and ulna, close to the radial bone.)

This point on the right wrist is the same as point 4 of circuit 13 against eczema.

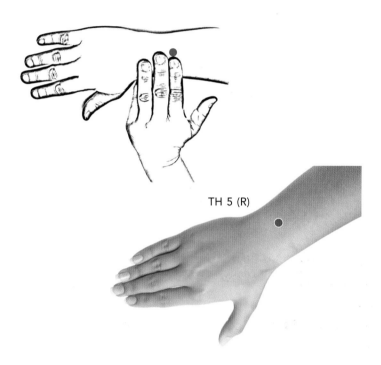

TH 5 (R)

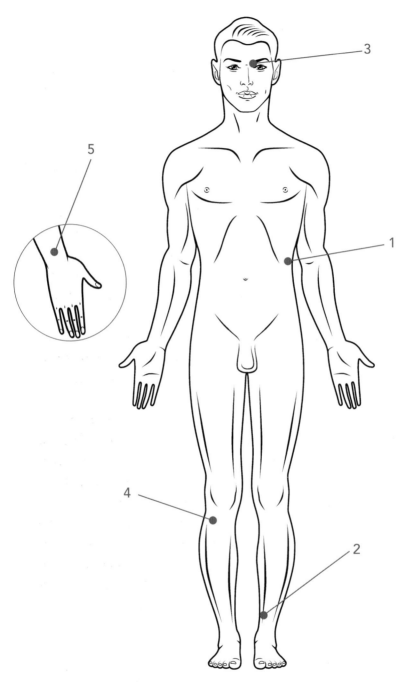

Circuit 20: Energizing the Solar Plexus

Against Impotence and Loss of Libido

Impotence is an issue that is often experienced as if it is the end of the world. It may generate self-deprecation, frustration, and depression. The person affected by this often loses his sense of self-worth and feels like a handicapped person whose life has been shattered; his partner bears the consequences as well, and the absence of this sexual dimension in a couple has a good chance of resulting in a painful breakup, except of course in the case of a very loving and stable relationship.

Impotence may appear without any objective or organic reason in a young man; in most cases, it is psychogenic, its source lying either in a simple single failure that has been experienced as a disaster, in ill-controlled latent guilt, or in the idealization of one's partner (the latter case possibly involving the confusion with the mother figure and thus resulting in a profound, unconscious sentiment of guilt).

In the case of an older person, impotence is experienced as the beginning of a decline in function; organic causes (high blood pressure, diabetes, and so forth) are responsible for it, although a significant psychological part remains.

The loss of libido, whether feminine or masculine, can be considered a lesser degree of impotence; understandably, it can be difficult to live with, particularly as it is often associated with a depressive state. Premature ejaculation could be considered as a lesser form of impotence as well; this issue is clearly liable to be a source of trouble.

The following circuit may prove very effective in all the above-mentioned situations, except in the cases of serious organic causes, which do not constitute the majority of such cases. This circuit should always be preceded by the circuits against fear (3), sometimes those against obsession (4) and depression (1); the next chapter will deal with this.

Point I: Liver 8 (Left)

(At the medial end of the left flexed knee crease, in a depression anterior to the tendons of semimembranosus and semitendinosus muscles.)

This point is located at the inner end of the crease of the flexed left knee, in a depression just in front of the tendons.

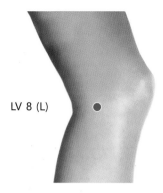

LV 8 (L)

Point 2: Spleen 10 (Left)

(On the inner left thigh, five centimeters above the inferior extremity of the femur.)

On the inside of your left knee, feel the big bony protuberance at the lower end of your thigh bone. Proceed upward along your thigh for about five centimeters, then press deeply. You can't get it wrong, as this point is very sensitive most of the time. This point is familiar to us; it is the same as point 2 of circuit 9 for restoring the yin/yang balance.

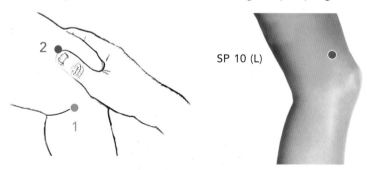

SP 10 (L)

Point 3: Gall Bladder 38 (Right)

(On the right ankle, about 8 cm above the tip of the lateral malleolus, on the anterior border of the fibula.)

Point 3 is located on the outside of your lower leg, about four finger-widths above the protruding end of the fibula. This point is symmetrical to point 4 of circuit 16 for energizing the colon.

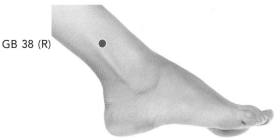

GB 38 (R)

Point 4: Kidney 3 (Left)

(On the left ankle in the depression between the medial malleolus and the Achilles tendon, level with the tip of the medial malleolus.)

This point is located on the inside of the left ankle, in the depression between the protruding lower end of the tibia and the Achilles tendon, level with the tip of the protrusion. This point is the same as point 3 of circuit 18 for stimulating creativity.

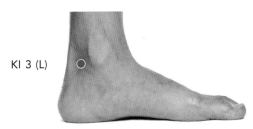

KI 3 (L)

Point 5: Governing Vessel 23

(From the anterior hairline follow the sagittal line of the skull back until a depression is felt at the anterior fontanel.)

We are familiar with this point in a depression on the midline of the skull.

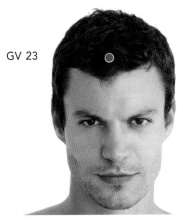

GV 23

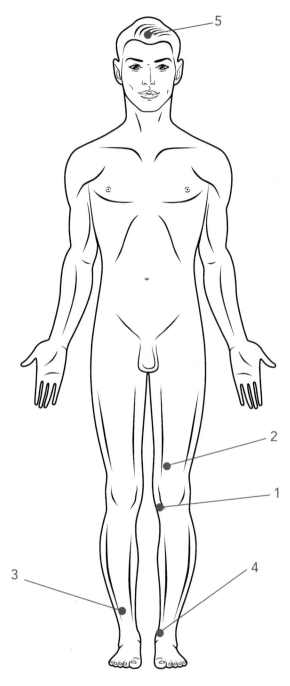

Circuit 21: Against Impotency and Loss of Libido

Circuit 22

Re-centering and Fostering Intuition

This book originally dealt only with the previously introduced 21 circuits. After a certain time, I began to suspect that a last circuit held enormous importance: it helps in finalizing the work that has been done by the other circuits and it re-centers the different "layers of energy" that surround our physical body. In this manner, this circuit enhances our intuitive abilities, hence its interest as an additional circuit.

Circuit 22 assists us in finding our way whenever we feel confused and are in need of being "re-centered." Insights and solutions to our current issues will thus be made possible.

Point 1: Conception Vessel 5

(On the midline, midway between the umbilicus and the superior part of the pubic bone.)

This point is located on the center axis of the body, midway between the navel and the top part of the pubic bone.

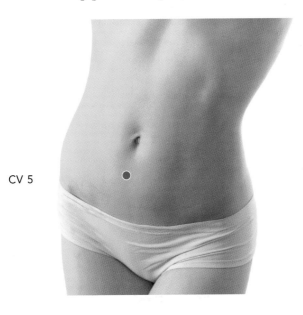

CV 5

Point 2: Governing Vessel 23

(From the anterior hairline follow the sagittal line of the skull back until a depression is felt at the anterior fontanel.)

We are familiar with this point, which corresponds to the anterior fontanel.

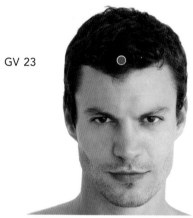

GV 23

Point 3: Spleen 6 (Left)

(On the internal side of the left ankle, 5 cm directly above the tip of the medial malleolus on the posterior border of the tibia.)

We have met with this point on several occasions already, particularly when dealing with negativity (point 1 in circuit 2 against negativity). It is situated on the inner side of the left ankle, about five centimeters above the prominence at the lower end of the tibia (larger lower leg bone).

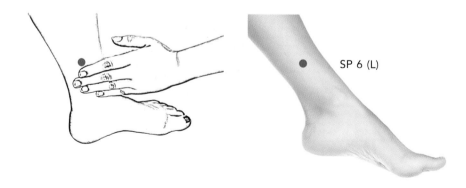

SP 6 (L)

Point 4: Stomach 36 (Right)

(At the crest and to the external side of the right tibia just below the kneecap.)

This point is well known to us by now, just below the right kneecap.

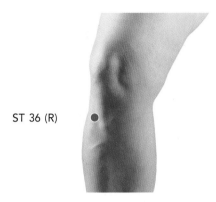

ST 36 (R)

Point 5: Urinary Bladder 67 (Left)

(Lateral aspect of the left little toe, 0.1 cm proximal to the corner of the nail.)

To locate this point, firmly hold your left little toe between the thumb and the second finger of your hand; carefully place your thumb upon the last phalanx, just before the corner of the nail and press firmly. This is symmetrical to point 1 of circuit 3 against anxiety.

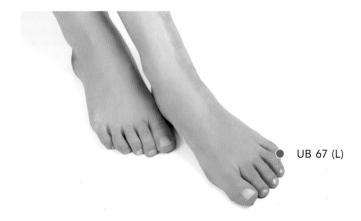

UB 67 (L)

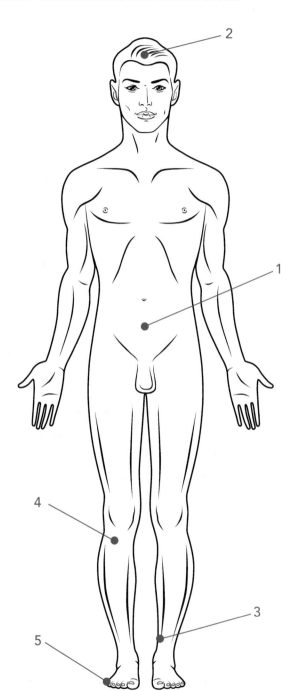

Circuit 22: Re-centering and Fostering Intuition

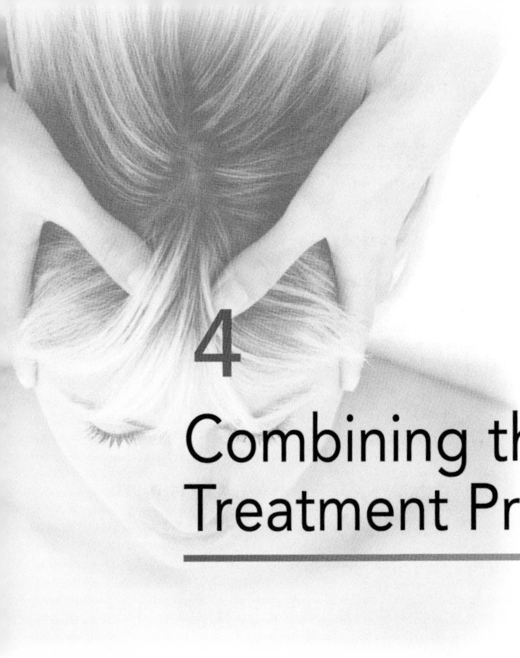

4
Combining the Circuits: Treatment Protocols

Miracles happen to those who believe in them.

BERNARD BERENSON

This chapter presents seven protocols made up of combinations of the circuits that are particularly effective for specific conditions. These protocols correspond to the most common emotional situations I have dealt with in my practice over the years:

+ Distress
+ Depression
+ Panic
+ Obsession
+ Jitters
+ Obesity
+ Hyper-emotionality

Before introducing the different protocols, I want to point out that outcomes are influenced by our beliefs; having faith in our wishes and projects has an effect on causality and constitutes a determining factor regarding a future achievement. In other words, the universe seems to not question, but respond to our demands.

It is often said that prayer should be a "thank you" instead of a request, as though what we wish for is already there; this is a good way to express our trust in the universe and to shut out any idea of doubt and failure. A strong affirmation infused with confidence is what we need; we want to concentrate on the result we wish for as though it is already present.

Scientists in the United States have worked with statistics and reached the conclusion that sick people who have no doubt that they will recover have a significantly higher chance of getting better than those who have given up all hope. Even more mind-boggling is that, according to Dr. Deepak Chopra, the well-known American endocrinologist and specialist in Ayurvedic medicine, a doctor's personal belief in his patient's recovery is a major factor: patients whose recovery was considered possible by their doctors did, in reality, recover more quickly and effectively than those who were thought of as lost causes by the medical staff (even though, of course, no opinion in those matters was ever voiced).

To sum up, it seems more and more certain that we affect all that happens to us, and that the will of our intentions does act on probability.

All these remarks corroborate the fact that, to make absolutely sure that we obtain satisfactory results with the different protocols, which deal with emergency situations, we have to believe in their efficacy. The point here is not to produce a placebo effect but to use the full force of our mind. Our thoughts have an extraordinary power that can affect our reality, provided they are given energy and channeled into a clear scenario.

I also want to emphasize that the earlier these protocols are used, the more effective they are: don't wait until you are completely imbalanced and don't wait for negative energies to accumulate. If an unpleasant remark or a disastrous meeting has left you emotionally shaken, it is a good idea to immediately do the Hyper-emotionality Protocol. The problem will be solved within five minutes, whereas not dealing with it on the spot will probably make of this new issue an unwelcome addition to a heap of already existing difficulties. The more negative we are, the more we feel threatened by anxiety, anguish, or panic.

While five point touch therapy can certainly take care of those emotional states, isn't it better for us to be proactive and avoid those destructive emotions? Just keep in mind that PBA may be used anywhere without people around you noticing what you are doing.

The name of each protocol is followed by the circuits that compose it; when circuits are shown in parentheses, that indicates they are optional additions, to be used if the conditions they relate to are also part of the present situation.

Distress Protocol

Circuits 10, 2, 1, 4, 3, 6, 7

This protocol will be of a great help in case of a major crisis or of an unexpected catastrophe, such as an accident, a piece of disastrous news, a sudden break up, or an unforeseen loss.

Being able to handle a challenging situation does not mean being indifferent to it; it means being better equipped to handle the crisis. As I often say to those of my patients who have just lost a loved one: "I'm not removing your sorrow; I can't do that, but what I can do for you is to give you the means to cope with the circumstances and to restore your potential for self-defense or survival."

If some Rescue Remedy (one of the Bach flower remedies) is available, you may place five drops of it under the tongue. This is not indispensable, but it will help with the process of "letting go" that we want to achieve with the action of the circuits.

Then, one after the other, apply the following circuits: 10, 2, 1, 4, 3, 6, 7. Repeat each of these operations three times. Circuit 10 deals with anger; circuit 2 with negativity; circuit 1 with depression; circuit 3 with fear; circuit 6 clears the "scars" left by previous trauma; circuit 7 restores the fundamental vibration.

As early as circuit 3, you will start to feel the tensions dissolving. If you are helping someone, you'll observe his face relax. Still, the protocol should be done in its totality, or, at least through circuit 7.

As we are dealing here with a serious situation, it is likely that the circuits will have to be reapplied after a few hours, and then a few days later. It probably won't be necessary to apply *all* the circuits though, especially circuit number 6 (the one that resets the "blown fuses").

When negativity and depression are retreating, you may do without the corresponding circuits. Depending on the person's progress, the protocol can be reduced, so that, after some time, it may be limited to only circuits 2, 3, and 7. There's no strict rule, as everything depends on the patient's reaction. If you sense diffidence, do not hesitate to use the muscle testing described in chapter 2; think, or tell the person you are helping to think, "I need (the specific) circuit," then check the reaction. Circuit number 4 against obsessions could be very useful here as well, if you feel that the patient's issue tends to become obsessive. Here again, muscle testing can prove worthwhile.

As a beginner, you may feel unsure of what you are doing and afraid to make a mistake, but please understand that applying the circuit against depression (or any other emotional state) when the patient does not need it expressly will produce *no* negative effect. On the other hand, *not* applying a circuit that is needed is definitely bound to make the whole process lose its efficacy.

All this is really not as difficult as it may look; sheer common sense, a reasonable sense of observation, and carefully listening to the patient are what it takes, and the muscle testing is there to confirm that you are on the right track. Nevertheless, in case of an extreme situation, or if you perceive too little progress, don't hesitate to see or recommend a doctor.

Remember that it's not up to you to advise the cessation of a medical treatment (such as an antidepressant): only the patient's doctor has authority in that matter. While the regular and systematic use of PBA definitely helps a person to do without or to stop using antidepressants before any chemical dependence occurs, keep in mind that the decision does not belong to you.

Please do not forget your "neutral shield" (see the fourth rule in chapter 6) every time you have to deal with extreme negativity; also carefully wash your hands after a session, for at least thirty seconds. You won't be of any use to your patient if you absorb all her negativity.

CASE STUDY
Numbness after a Shock

Thirty-five-year-old Camille came to consult me. Her partner and father of their little Ben had just left them, without any sign or warning. Some days before she came, he had left home and only called briefly to make sure Ben was coping well.

Camille had no clue at all about the reasons he deserted them; things had seemed to be fine. What worried me was Camille's response: "This is strange; I feel as though I have no sensitivity at all. I know I should feel bad and sad, yet I seem to feel nothing."

I'm familiar with this type of reaction, when the person seems to be handling the situation, yet can't feel anything. The violence of the shock causes the brain to produce an apparent insensitivity, which is supposed to give protection. I have often heard people who have just lost a loved one say that they feel totally numb; this apparent lack of "normal" reaction makes them feel very guilty. But I'm aware that this numbness, which can be compared to an anesthesia of the mind, won't last forever and that the risk of a major breakdown is very real.

Camille's lack of reaction pinpointed the seriousness of the situation. I selected the Distress Protocol. Camille's tears began to flow at the end of circuit 3; they were the signal that she was starting to release her bottled-up tensions. When the session was over, she was far more relaxed, as though she had been relieved of a terrible weight; she said: 'What you did there was pure magic." Her situation did not change, but her approach to it did. She was then capable of coping with it without having to hide behind a wall of tense coldness and aloofness. She no longer had the need for a system of artificial protection.

I sincerely believe that the preventive use of psycho-bio-acupressure prevented Camille from spiraling downward and experiencing a severe depression. Happily, she consulted me before that happened, at the advice of a friend. She did not regret it for a second. I taught Camille how to apply the circuits herself, and soon she could ably handle her circumstances. The Distress Protocol is an extremely powerful tool that I have used over and over again with the same success.

Depression Protocol

Circuits 2, 1, 3, (4), (5), (6), 7, (9)

We mentioned the principal signs of depression when we studied its corresponding circuit (circuit 1). Self-sabotage is always a possibility that needs to be checked; you may want to use some Rescue Remedy, which helps to dissolve tensions, but is not indispensable in this case.

Systematically apply the following circuits: 2, 1, 3, and 7 (against negativity, depression, and fear, and to restore the fundamental vibration). Depending on the case, before circuit 7, you may add circuit 4 (if obsession is detected), circuit 5 (if hyper-emotionality is perceived as excessive), and circuit 6 (if there's a serious psychological trauma at the source of the depression). Always end the session with circuit 7 and, possibly, circuit 9 for restoring the yin/yang balance, which puts the finishing touch to the whole process. This does not take as long as it looks.

Depending on the progress made, these circuits may have to be done every day, and then every two days, then again every three days. You may progressively do without circuits 1 and 2.

Once again, *do not* risk anything and remain cautious when dealing with depression. Do not hesitate to seek professional advice. If you have morbid thoughts or if you are aware that the person you are helping is having morbid thoughts, don't wait to see a doctor. The work you are doing in PBA will enhance the effects of the medical treatment and will help to make recovery happen sooner. Depression is too serious a problem to take any inconsiderate risk. Never deal with it by yourself. Seek professional help.

Depression is not age-related; it may occur in teenagers, and even children and babies. Because a child or a teenager has different ways to express depression, verbal expression won't usually be your clue, but the child's behavior, at school or at home, will indicate that something is definitely wrong.

CASE STUDY
Coping with Bullying

Amber was twelve years old. She was approaching puberty, her body was changing, and she had skin problems. It is common knowledge that this time of life is not smooth: leaving childhood behind often means leaving a worry-free era behind, and the inevitable physical change is frequently a source of anxiety.

Amber was stressed out and constantly tearful. For two years, a girl her own age had severely bullied her at school. When she came to see me, Amber was in a different school, but she still saw this girl when she had her horse-riding classes, which she liked. However, having to be in the company of this bully twice a week terrified her to the extent that a phobia developed. Amber had become unable to think of anything else but this girl and was seriously thinking of putting an end to her horse riding, though she was very good at it.

I applied the following circuits: 2 against negativity, 1 against depression, 3 against fear, 4 for dealing with obsessions, 6 for removing energetic scars left by previous trauma, and 7 for restoration of the fundamental vibration.

Amber got better very rapidly; by the second session, I only needed to apply circuit 5 against hyper-emotionality and circuit 9 for restoring the yin/yang balance.

Amber decided to carry on with her horse-riding classes; the best part was that she became almost indifferent to the other girl's bullying and that her school results considerably improved. PBA solved her problem in two weeks.

This protocol can also be very helpful for a baby who cries constantly, cannot go to sleep, and suffers from chronic colic. This is particularly true for those babies whose delivery was long and difficult (requiring forceps or cesarean section). It is all the more true if the baby had to stay in an incubator for a while. These babies have perceived and absorbed their mother's energy of panic during delivery, or even occasionally, the panic of the medical staff; unable to analyze this panic, they have developed their own panic of being brought into the world. Besides, they have been forced to leave the comfort zone of the womb in rather rough conditions and very often have lost contact with their mother for the few hours or even the few days following their birth. As a result, they have not only the panic of being born, but the panic of abandonment as well. Not to mention the terror of being assaulted if they have been handled a bit roughly.

In his book, *Rediscovering Real Medicine: The New Horizons of Homeopathy,* Jean Emilger quite rightly insists on the importance of taking these babies to a good osteopath, who specializes in cranial matters and who can manipulate the cranium bones to their original position. (This is all the more necessary if forceps or spoons have been involved.) This manipulation will allow the liquids in which the brain floats to regain a free flow.

It is also indispensable to apply the circuits against depression and fear (1 and 3), as well as circuit 6 that clears the energetic scars and circuit 7 to restore the fundamental vibration. The result will be instant. The very day of the treatment, the baby will be able to sleep peacefully and behave normally. It might be useful sometimes to add the circuit for the colon in case of colic.

The younger a child is, the more effective PBA is; the child harbors no doubt during the session and is not over-rational and skeptical regarding the efficacy of what is being done to him. His mind does not interfere with a million questions; it is not locked into a single perspective and this definitely helps with quicker results.

Needless to say, we must be extremely gentle and cautious when working on a baby: a baby's limbs and toes are tiny, her skin is highly sensitive, and one must clearly exert great circumspection when applying pressure. Pressure must be very light, and stop immediately the moment the baby's skin becomes a little whiter or paler. Once these precautions are taken, the results are astounding.

Panic Protocol

Circuits 2, 3, (6), 7, (9)

Anxiety is clearly difficult to live with: it involves a constant sensation of having a weight on the chest, and occasionally the sensation of a painful burn at the level of the solar plexus.

A constant lump in one's throat, achingly clenched jaws, endless palpitations, and a throbbing migraine that induces tension in the cervical vertebrae: these symptoms signal that anxiety is on its way to becoming a chronic problem. Life soon grows intolerable and psychosomatic reactions begin to take a number of guises, such as stomach ulcer, psoriasis attacks, or even cancers. Anxiety must be tracked down and treated as soon as it is detected.

Panic is a more transitory state: it takes the form of amplified anxiety; it is paralyzing and causes nausea, cold sweats, and the inability to do normal activities of life such as boarding a plane or driving a car. Panic is terrifying, as it induces an overwhelming feeling of imminent death.

PBA will be of great help here. The protocol to be used is circuits 2, 3, 7 (against negativity and fear, and restoring the fundamental vibration), and, if needed, circuit 9 to restore the yin/yang balance. If it seems as though the person has experienced a major psychological shock, squeeze circuit 6 for removing energetic scars between circuits 3 and 7, but do this only once, as this circuit is usually definitively and immediately effective.

CASE STUDY
Obsessive Fear

Alexandra had convinced herself that she did not know how to take proper care of her eight-month-old baby.

Little Sam was not a healthy feeder, to say the least, and his mother was absolutely terrified because he strongly reminded her of her own sister who almost died of anorexia when she was eighteen.

Naturally, this tendency seemed to worsen rapidly. Baby Sam systematically turned his little head sideways as soon as a spoon or a bottle filled his field of vision; each meal was a nightmare and Alexandra could not help but be apprehensive at nursing time. Things grew so bad that she did not even feel like going home after work even though she cherished her baby. The woman who provided child care during the day for Sam had told her that the child fed normally at her place; knowing this was an extra source of guilt and anxiety for Alexandra, who soon developed a deep sense of inadequacy as a mother.

During our session, Alexandra talked extensively about the baby and her own fears. Anorexia was clearly becoming an obsession and sleep was a long-past luxury. I applied circuits 2, 3, 7, and added circuit 4 against obsessions. I recommended that she do the circuit against fear on herself each day before leaving for work and before feeding Sam. I also instructed her to do the whole protocol—circuits 2, 3, and 7—every morning when she got up. We agreed that I would see the baby in four days' time in order to restore the balance of his energies and look for the cause of his feeding problem.

Three days later, Alexandra cancelled her appointment: Samuel had started feeding normally. His mother was elated. Her negative energies (fear and obsession) were gone and little Sam definitely felt safe again.

This anecdote calls for a couple of remarks:

1. Anxiety is highly contagious: baby Sam felt his mother's anguish and reacted by stopping feeding, hence the importance of our "neutral shield."
2. Protocols are totally flexible: they are not subject to rules and can be modified according to your own assessment. With Alexandra, I chose to add the circuit against obsession to the classic Panic Protocol.

All this is common sense and intuition. I also remember the case of little Cynthia.

CASE STUDY
Panic Attacks

Cynthia was Australian and had gone to New Caledonia with her family for the holidays. Before leaving Sydney, her parents were unaware of a serious issue: their daughter was subject to terrible panic attacks on a plane; the flight proved an absolute nightmare. The child even ran to the plane door and tried to open it. Her breathing was difficult and during the whole journey she was either livid or very flushed and, in both cases, totally terrified. The idea of flying back home was enough to spoil everyone's vacation.

One more time, PBA proved remarkably useful: I applied the Panic Protocol and taught Cynthia's parents circuit 3 against fear, anxiety, and panic, asking them to apply it every day until D-day at the airport. A few days later, an email let me know that the journey back home had been without incident: Cynthia had been a little tense but there was a world of difference from the first trip.

Obsession Protocol
Circuits (10), 4, 3, 2, 7, (9)

Most of us have experienced obsession at least once: a financial problem, a breakup, or the unexpected verdict of the weighing scales might have triggered obsession at some level or another. If we realize that we are finding it impossible to think of anything other than our current preoccupation, and if we have to acknowledge the fact that we have become incapable of listening to anyone or of concentrating on anything, that is an indication that it is high time we apply this protocol. The urgency is the more real given that brooding over the same problem is the best way to block our capacity to realize an answer to the issue. Fixating on a problem cripples us by limiting our vision.

Hence, this protocol includes the following circuits: 4 against obsession; 3, because clearly obsession produces the fear of not finding a solution; 2, because fear causes negativity; and 7 (and possibly 9) to finish. In the days after beginning the protocol, and depending on progress, you can use circuit 4 for dealing with obsessions more particularly; fear and negativity will be taken care of.

CASE STUDY
Identifying Obsessive Behavior

A patient of mine, a young woman whose fiancé had broken up with her, could not cope with her situation, and after her third session with me, no significant change was observed.

I had applied the circuits against depression, fear, and negativity, the one against hyper-emotionality, and the one that clears the scars caused by previous trauma. Still nothing had changed. I had made sure that there was no self-sabotage involved. Eventually I began to have serious doubts myself until I realized that her problem had become an obsession that circuit 4 could perfectly take care of. A single session that included this Obsession Protocol was enough to unblock the situation.

CASE STUDY
Moving Past Obsession and Anger

Among many stories, I remember the case of a schoolteacher who experienced nothing but difficulties and delays with the building of his new house: his first. Contractor had gone bankrupt and left the building site in a mess; the second one proved no better; meanwhile, problems with his bank loans were becoming overwhelming because the first contractor had been dishonest. Construction deadlines were long past and my dismayed patient found himself in a problematical position: he had to pay back his loan as well as pay for extra house rent he had not been expecting.

Needless to say, the problem had developed into a real obsession; his work at school began to suffer, not to mention his family life. I applied the Obsession Protocol, and before that, circuit 10 to deal with the suppressed anger that was inevitable and strong. My patient immediately recovered; I taught him the protocol to help him along. Without it, I'm positive that he was heading toward a major nervous breakdown.

Jitters Protocol

Circuits 2, 3, 5, 8

Jitters typically occur before an exam when we suddenly find ourselves incapable of thinking coherently or of giving relevant answers, or when we have to ask our bank manger for a much-needed overdraw; our unstable emotional state makes us inarticulate and unable to present our case as we should. In other words, jitters are a special kind of panic that deprives us of all our resources during a driving test or a first date. Situations in which we find ourselves deprived of our usual means of articulate communication are endless, but their consequences may definitely be disastrous.

Whatever the case, the Jitters Protocol is extremely effective; it had gained so much recognition in Nouméa that I used to devote an entire week to high school students just before their final exams for graduation. As I told them, I clearly could not help them pass if they had not studied, but I certainly could do something about that paralyzing fear and help them deal with the challenge.

This protocol is mainly constituted of circuits 2, 3, 5, and 8 (against negativity, fear, hyper-emotionality, plus the circuit that helps with expression). Please note that this protocol does not require circuits 7 or 9 for restoring the fundamental vibration and the yin/yang balance.

CASE STUDY
Public Speaking

Maurice had to present the annual report of the charity of which he was president as well as secretary. He was a volunteer for this job, which he took extremely seriously, so seriously in fact that the pressure was fast becoming unbearable, as were his sleepless nights.

Maurice could not help but be extremely apprehensive of the day he would have to present his report in public. He had never felt at ease when talking in front of a crowd and this had been a life-long issue: even speaking with a woman would scare him out of his wits when he was younger.

I applied the Jitters Protocol and taught him the four relevant circuits. I recommended that he do it every morning before and on his "D-day." A few days later, he called me to let me know that he had truly impressed his public and that those who had been aware of his previous difficulties congratulated him warmly for having done so well.

Each time I get similar news, I'm happy for two reasons: I feel happy for my patient and I feel happy to have another evidence of the efficacy of PBA as a life-altering method.

Obesity Protocol

Circuits (2), 4, 3, 5, 9

When applied every day, morning and night, this protocol can be of a great help to those with weight problems.

There are basically two main causes for a weight issue: in a minority of cases, there's an organic cause linked to an organ that works defectively; this is usually an endocrine gland such as the pituitary in the case of an adenoma, or the thyroid when it functions insufficiently. A number of other medical causes exist as well and generally need to be treated by mainstream medical methods. In those cases, this protocol becomes effective only once the organic cause has been treated.

Nonetheless, a psychosomatic cause is at the source of the majority of cases and corresponds to a system of defense. Basically, we put on weight because we are scared: as already mentioned, one of our primordial fears is starvation. So each time we feel anxiety, our most primitive brain (reptilian), which contains the whole of the memory of our species, does not analyze the real source of anxiety, but gives our body the order to gorge on food as if the risk of starvation was real. The result is of course weight gain.

The fear of being attacked may also be responsible for those extra pounds: our primitive brain determines that wrapping our body in fat layers protects us against the world. This is the reason why yo-yo situations are common: a slimming diet makes us thinner; then our anxiety reappears, because we feel unprotected at some deep level; the result is that somehow we end up putting on weight again. Paradoxically, another fear that causes obesity is the fear of being sexually attractive, hence an unconscious desire to become physically unappealing.

The protocol is circuits 4, 3, 5, and 9. It has to be done twice a day: upon getting up in the morning and before the evening meal. Circuit 4 takes care of obsession, as a weight problem is always linked to obsession; circuit 3 deals with the latent fear mentioned above; circuit 5 deals with hyper-emotionality, which is bound to exist in this case. Circuit 9 restores the yin/yang balance as well as our metabolism.

In the beginning, circuit 2 against negativity may also be applied, as negativity is obviously related to the self-image of the overweight person; this circuit is to be done first. Make sure to look for signs of depression and add circuit 1 if they are present.

As things start to get better, circuits 5 and 9 will remain, and then only circuit 9.

Hyper-emotionality Protocol

Circuits 5, 7

This protocol is appropriate for the numerous cases when you feel not exactly anxious, but still hyper-sensitive. Compared to the previously discussed situations, hyper-sensitivity may seem not earnest enough to deserve attention, but blushing furiously or crying uncontrollably can be socially mortifying. It can cause real difficulties in relationships, and some of us may find it a bit ludicrous to be fully grown up and unable to control copious tears at, say, the happy ending of a romantic comedy.

On the other hand, some of us can also find this quite charming. However, for those who consider it discomfiting to be unable to control their hyper-sensitivity, the protocol that can take care of this little problem consists of circuits 5 against hyper-emotionality and 7 to restore the fundamental vibration. These circuits should be done regularly, morning and evening, for a few weeks. As soon as you sense that an embarrassing situation is coming, you may preemptively and discreetly apply circuit 5.

Using the Protocols

Let me take the opportunity now to remind you that these protocols, particularly the Jitters and Hyper-emotionality Protocols, can really be done anywhere without attracting uncalled-for attention. All it takes is keeping in mind the different points of acupressure; the rest follows easily. This aspect of PBA, together with its great effectiveness, is exactly what makes this method truly exciting. It is flexible and efficient.

At this stage, it is possible that, although I did my best to introduce the circuits and protocols as clearly as I could, some of you may wonder about your abilities and let doubt enter your minds, such as: "Will I be able, even with the help of the muscle testing, to identify what state I'm in, or to help someone else? What kind of consequence will there be if I'm not correct in selecting the relevant circuits?"

I want to reassure you by talking a little bit about the workshops I conduct. The energetic states of the participants are obviously all different. Before starting the work, I test each of them: some are depressed, others anguished, or emotionally very fragile; some are okay and are there to enrich their knowledge and to learn how to keep negative emotions in check.

To begin with, I teach everyone how to apply the nine main circuits and I write the details on a board. Then, each participant tries to apply the circuits on a fellow participant and to locate the different points on his or her own body. In the end, everyone has experienced the circuits on their own body. I won't detail the whole development of the workshops here; suffice it to say that, at the end, I test everyone again. The energetic state of each one is perfectly balanced.

From this we can draw the conclusion that a number of people have "received" circuits they obviously did not need, as they were not particularly depressed or anxious. The fact of having "received" circuits they did not expressly require did not disturb them at all. It has been shown again and again that it is totally safe to apply a circuit that does not correspond exactly to what a person's current energetic state exactly requires.

Therefore, when you are unsure about which circuits to select, you should just apply the nine main ones. It would be truly a shame not to do a much-needed circuit just because of an incorrect diagnosis. Of course, it will take a little longer to do all nine, but at least you'll be quite certain to have forgotten nothing and to have achieved a well-balanced energetic level.

As you gain experience and feel more confident about what you feel and do, you will really learn how to respond exactly to what your energy state requires. But, in the beginning, there's absolutely no harm in applying the nine main circuits. Do not hesitate to apply circuit 10 against suppressed anger if improvement seems a bit too slow.

During the workshops, people often inquire about the length of time required between the application of a circuit and the following one. In case of an emergency, when fast action is crucial, there's no need to pause between two circuits because clearly the priority is to get rid of an emotionally unbearable situation.

Nevertheless, if you have time and find yourself in a calm and quiet environment, you may want to allow some minutes between two circuits in order to fully appreciate their effects and feel a deep relaxation state progressively developing.

You may want to listen to some relaxing music or do some quiet breathing so that this energetic "recharge" becomes a moment of true happiness. Doing this each morning is the ideal arrangement; otherwise, devoting some time to the circuits on the weekends will greatly contribute to your wellbeing and clear negative energies.

The following table summarizes all of the protocols. Each circuit should be performed in the order shown in the table, from top to bottom. The symbol "X" indicates the circuits that must be included, while the symbol "( )" indicates optional circuits.

RECAPITULATION OF THE PROTOCOLS

	Distress	Depression	Panic	Hyper-emotional	Obsession	Jitters	Obesity
Circuit 10: Against Suppressed Anger	( )	( )			( )		
Circuit 2: Against Negativity	X	X	X	( )	X	X	X
Circuit 1: Against Depression	X	X		( )			( )
Circuit 3: Against Fear, Anxiety, and Panic	X	X	X	( )	X	X	X
Circuit 4: Dealing with Obsessions	( )	( )	( )	( )	X	( )	X
Circuit 5: Against Hyper-Emotionality	( )	( )	( )	X		X	X
Circuit 6: Removing Scars from Our Energetic System	X	X	( )				( )
Circuit 7: Restoring the Fundamental Vibration	X		X	X	X		( )
Circuit 9: Restoring the Yin/Yang Balance		( )		( )	( )		X
Circuit 8: Enhancing Expression						X	

5
Glossary of Conditions and Recommended Protocols

In this chapter you will find a glossary of the most common emotional issues and psychosomatic diseases and their corresponding protocols. My experience in dealing with these conditions allows me in many cases to recommend both an initial protocol as well as a "maintenance" one to be used once things start to get better; a "maintenance" protocol is a "light" protocol to be used in the second phase only. The circuits shown in brackets are optional: their use depends on the context.

If possible, respect the sequence of application of circuits that is provided; I have experimented with different possibilities for a long time to make absolutely sure that the ones I present here are the most effective.

While the following list is not exhaustive, your common sense can help you deal with the situations that have not been described. The descriptions of the 22 circuits will assist you.

Let me remind you of some basic precautions: before applying the circuits, remove your watch or anything that contains batteries (remote, car keys, mobile phone). Check to be sure you are not dealing with a case of self-sabotage: use the muscle testing to verify that you may safely begin the session. If you are helping somebody else, make sure you build your "neutral shield" (per the fourth rule in chapter 6) at the beginning of the session, and wash your hands at the end of it.

Abandonment

Circuits (10), 2, 1, 3, 4, 5, 6, 7

Abandonment is a very common issue and is liable to have massive consequences for the affected person. Prevention is definitely crucial in order to avoid future emotional damage.

This issue may have different causes: the departure of a loved one is generally the most common occurrence. Nonetheless, it is frequent for a child to feel abandoned by his or her mother, whether at the birth of a new baby brother or sister, or when she goes back to work a few weeks after his or her own birth. Among common causal events, a parents' divorce may figure as well. A loss can be perceived as a desertion.

Whatever the reason, the person who suffers from this feeling of abandonment will do everything to prevent the repetition of a similar situation in the future. It can result in being incapable of making a romantic commitment, as commitment means the possibility of being deserted. Or a person could get involved in endless impossible affairs, always selecting emotionally unavailable partners, because the unconscious mind feels safe only when the situation holds no promise of the relationship going to a deeper level.

Make sure that you check for depression (circuit 1), as there is a high probability it will be present, and that you clearly acknowledge the risks it involves; also check if there's any suppressed anger (circuit 10); if there is, it has to be cleared, particularly in the case of an adult who has been deserted by a lover.

In a situation of abandonment there can be a high possibility of a destructive act against oneself or the partner (particularly in the case of young people); be extremely careful in such situations. Never hesitate to ask for professional advice if the situation does not improve rapidly.

Circuit 2 is obviously needed as well because of negativity, as are circuit 3 against fear and circuit 4 for dealing with obsession. Circuit 6 has to be done on the first session because the violence of the shock has most probably made "the fuses blow."

As a maintenance protocol once the depressive state starts to decrease, circuit 1 can be left off; same is true with circuit 3 when fear diminishes. Circuit 6 is really only needed the first time. Circuits 2, 4, 5 (against negativity, obsession, hyper-emotionality), and, of course, 7 (to restore the primordial vibration) need to be done for some time.

Accident

Circuits 2, 1, 3, (4), 5, 6, 7

In this kind of circumstance, when acting without hesitation is essential, the Distress Protocol should be done immediately (see chapter 4). If some Rescue Remedy is available, it will increase the effects of the circuits.

CASE STUDY
Using Distress Protocol After an Accident

A young mother of a six-year-old had been a participant in one of my workshops; some time afterward, her daughter had an accident while riding an all-terrain vehicle, in which she was very roughly ejected on the roadside; it is easy to imagine the state of panic in so young a child.

Her mother immediately applied the Distress Protocol. Some days later, when she brought the little girl to my practice, I found no trace of negative emotion in the child's energetic system, although some could have been expected after such an accident. The little girl was absolutely fine, and once again, the efficacy of this protocol had proved to be very high.

Alopecia or Hair Loss

See Scalp Diseases.

Anger

Circuits 10, 2, 1, 4, 3, 6, 7

Anger is a negative emotional state, which, if left uncontrolled, can hinder judgment and affect behavior.

Anguish

Circuits 2, 3, (6), 7

As with anxiety, the context will make it clear which circuits need to be associated with the main circuit, which is circuit 3 (against fear, anxiety, and panic). For more details, please see the Panic Protocol in chapter 4.

Anorexia

Circuits 2, 1, 3, 4, 5, 6, 7

We are not referring here to common loss of appetite, the one that is related to pressure and fatigue, but to real anorexia. Its treatment will benefit from a lengthy application of the Depression Protocol twice a day. However, if the symptom is diagnosed as actual anorexia nervosa, then do not limit the treatment to PBA. Seek professional advice as psychotherapy or even a stay in the hospital might be necessary. Anorexia is a major issue; be very cautious when dealing with it. PBA can be helpful as an accompaniment to other treatment in order to accelerate its effects.

Anxiety

Circuits 3, 2, 5, 7

The specific circuit against anxiety is circuit 3 (see chapter 2). A slight anxiety, such as can be felt when one is expecting the result of a university exam, can be treated with circuit 3 only, likewise for that feeling of apprehension that appears when we are not sure about getting some refreshing sleep after a long and exhausting day.

Depending on the case, circuit 3 may be used in conjunction with other circuits. Circuit 2 is certainly needed if anxiety is accompanied by negativity; likewise for circuit 5, if there's hyper-emotionality, and circuit 7 in order to restore the fundamental vibration of all the energetic centers. Do not hesitate to refer to the Panic Protocol (chapter 4).

Apathy

Circuits 2 , 1, 3, 6, 7

Apathy or abulia is characterized by a total lack of desire and motivation, which we know is symptomatic of depression; refer to the Depression Protocol in chapter 4.

Asthma

Circuits (2), 12, (1), 3, (4), 5, (6), 7

In some cases, asthma may be related to allergies. In such cases, PBA will have little impact: when the percentage of antibodies is very high and when the substance (the antigen) that has caused this proliferation is again present, a conflict usually emerges that will be expressed in the form of an asthma attack. We cannot do much then, except work upon the anxiety that has caused it. (Do circuit 3 against fear.)

On the other hand, an attack may be directly stress-induced. This is frequently the case with children who are apprehensive about a school test: the attack happens right on time. In this case, PBA can either abort the asthma attack or decrease its intensity.

Priority is to be given to circuit 12, which restores the ether element; we saw that stress was responsible for its "disconnection." This should be accompanied by circuit 3 against fear, circuit 5 against hyper-emotionality, and circuit 7 for restoring the fundamental vibration.

Depending on the preexisting state that might have increased the fragility of the subject, you'll decide whether to apply circuit 2 against negativity, circuit 1 against depression, circuit 6 to remove scars of previous trauma, or circuit 4 against obsessions.

Always be extremely vigilant and if things do not get better rapidly, consult a doctor immediately.

Bedwetting (Enuresis)

Circuits 2, 1, 3, 5, (6), 7, 15

This is another psychosomatic reaction to anxiety: the anxious child's unconscious mind wants to recreate the safe and reassuring warm environment he used to experience in the womb. (Amniotic liquid and urine share a very similar composition.) It is not surprising, therefore, that this protocol includes the circuits that deal with fear and depression. It is of crucial importance to end the session with circuit 15 to stimulate the bladder.

As a maintenance protocol, I recommend circuit 3 against fear and circuit 15 for the bladder to be done just before the child goes to bed.

Bulimia

Circuits 1, 2, 3, 4, 5, 6, 7, 9

This protocol concerns itself with the major kind of overeating that is accompanied by a systematic tendency to make oneself sick, and by the resulting and inevitable feelings of shame, guilt, and self-deprecation.

In the beginning, be careful to check for the presence of depression (addressed by circuit 1), which seems ineluctable. As a maintenance protocol, because of the almost inescapable obsession state, keep circuits 2, 3, 4, 7, and 9. Also take note of the presence in this protocol of circuit 9 that restores the yin/yang balance and thus acts upon metabolism.

Bullying

Circuits (10), 2, 1, 3, 4, 6, 7

A depressive and obsessive state constitutes the main element here, but suppressed anger may be present as well. This protocol must systematically be done as long as the situation in question lasts.

Chronic Fatigue (Asthenia)

Circuits 2, 1, 3, 7

This is not the common tiredness that emerges when we overwork. This refers to intense and lasting fatigue. Obviously, priority must be given to medical tests (biological and hormonal) in order to identify any organic cause.

Once the required medical tests have been done and come back clear, the possibility of a psychosomatic origin may be considered. In that case, refer to the Depression Protocol, as this kind of fatigue is an important symptom of depression. It could even be the only visible sign of a real depression that the subject is attempting to suppress. Even when the person deliberately ignores the seriousness of the situation, that does not mean that the issue is not real.

Colic in a Newborn

Circuits 3, 6, 7, 16

A newly born baby who suffers from colic is a scared baby. As mentioned before, the mother's pregnancy may have been psychologically or physically difficult, generating anxiety that may have been perceived and absorbed by the baby; this resulted in her own energetic imbalance. Another scenario is that problems occurring during delivery left the baby scared and scarred. This can be all the more the case if forceps were used (she might have sensed those as an act of aggression), or if a cesarean section was performed (a rough separation from the comfort of the womb and the reassuring maternal vibrations can certainly be experienced as highly traumatic). In all cases, panic occurred.

The following four circuits—3 against fear, 6 for removing scars left by previous trauma, 7 to restore the fundamental vibration, and especially 16 for energizing the colon—are highly effective; their results are very impressive with babies who had previously been crying all the time. Do not forget to be very cautious and delicate when applying pressure.

Colon Pathologies (Spasmodic or Functional) in an Adult

Circuits 2, (1), 3, (4), 5, 6, 7, 16

These conditions manifest as painful spasms of the large intestine. When no organic or parasitic cause can be found, they are generally related to an anxious personality.

This protocol naturally includes the circuits against negativity (2), fear (3), and hyper-emotionality (5), together with 16 for energizing the colon; we have to keep in mind that a possible depression or obsession can be present as well.

Conflicts

Circuits (10), 2, 1, 3, 4, (5), 6, 7

After a major conflict, there's a good chance of the person "blowing his or her fuses" to the point that the Panic Protocol is required.

A latent conflict, which has a lengthy duration, will benefit from a maintenance protocol of circuit 1 against depression and circuit 4 against obsession. So, as long as the conflict remains unresolved, apply these on a daily basis: circuit 2 against negativity, circuit 1 against depression, circuit 3 against fear, circuit 4 against obsession, and, lastly, circuit 7 for restoring the fundamental vibration.

Cystitis, Repetitive

Circuits (1), 2, 3, 4, 5, 6, 7, 15

See also Infections, Repetitive.

In such cases it is important to work on fears and guilt. For the first treatment, begin with circuit 1 against depression if signs of depression are detected, and with circuit 6 for removing scars of possible trauma. As a maintenance protocol, apply circuit 5 against hyper-emotionality, circuit 7 to restore the fundamental vibration, and circuit 15 for energizing the bladder.

Depression

Circuits 2, 1, 3, (4), (5), (6), 7, (9)

Depression concerns adults as well as children; please see the Depression Protocol in chapter 4.

Desire to Have a Baby

Circuits 2, 1, 4, 3, 5, 7, 9, 19

This desire can very easily grow into an obsession, hence the importance of circuit 4 for dealing with obsessions. The first time, also systematically apply circuits 1 and 2 (against depression and negativity), because the frustration of not having a baby is frequently connected with a feeling of guilt or self-deprecation, which in turn, can develop into a component of depression. Make sure that this protocol systematically ends with circuit 19 for energizing the sacral plexus, which will restore energy to the area that controls the ovaries and the uterus.

As a maintenance protocol, do circuit 4 on a daily basis: not letting go of the desire for a pregnancy can prevent a pregnancy from happening. I therefore recommend circuits 4, 7 (to restore the fundamental vibration), and 19 (to energize the sacral plexus), to be done every day.

Divorce, Separation

See Abandonment.

Dyslexia

Circuits 11, 2, (1), 3, 5, 8

Circuit 11 has proved to be of a major assistance in cases of dyslexia because it restores the energetic coordination between the right and the left hemispheres of the brain. The dyslexic child is clearly in pain; the following circuits can bring major relief: circuits 2, 3, and 5 (against negativity, fear, and hyper-emotionality). Circuit 1 against depression may prove useful as well (let's not forget that depressed children have their own way of expressing their depressive state). Always finish with circuit 8 for enhancing expression.

These circuits have to be done on a daily basis for several weeks; then, keep circuits 5 and 8 as a maintenance protocol. The child's progress will truly amaze any professionals she might be working with, who could benefit from systematically applying circuit 11 to restore the energetic coordination of the brain and circuit 8 to enhance expression at the beginning of each session. These circuits are easy to learn and take five minutes to be applied.

Ear Infections, Repetitive

Circuits 2, 3, 4, 5, 7, 8

See Infections, Repetitive.

Eczema

Circuits 2, 12, (1), 3, 5, (6), (4), 7, 13

When we studied circuit 13, we observed that eczema is *the* psychosomatic disease par excellence; it is related to suppressed anxiety, which has caused the ether element to be disconnected and caused the emergence of the energies of anguish and hyper-emotionality. The first days, don't hesitate to treat obsessions (circuit 4) or possibly depression (circuit 1).

As a maintenance protocol, I suggest circuits 12, 5, 7, and 13 (on a daily basis). If a depressive, obsessive, or negative component turns up again, add the corresponding circuits (1, 4, and 2).

In my daily practice, these protocols have proven to be really effective, notably on the eczema of newborn babies, which, I have no doubt, is almost totally related to fears that have been experienced in the womb or during delivery. Again, let us not forget that a child, even a newborn, can be affected by energies of depression and that, in that case, we may have to apply the corresponding circuit (1).

It is also a possibility that lactose intolerance causes eczema and we want to keep that in mind if the circuits produce no result. Nonetheless, I think that it is good to try this protocol before opting for a radical change in the baby's diet, or after a change of diet has given no result.

Dyshidrosis is one of the specific forms of eczema, which more particularly affects the hands, more rarely the feet, and causes the formation of intensely itchy little vesicles on the fingers and the palms (or toes and sole). These vesicles may burst and produce peeling of the skin. This disorder may be painful and is the sign of a very anxious character. The general protocol for eczema is effective in this and other specific kinds as well.

Exam Jitters

Circuits 2, 3, 5, 8

See Jitters Protocol in chapter 4.

Fear

Circuits 2, 3, (6), 7, (9)

See Panic Protocol in chapter 4.

Fears of the Newborn, Unexplained

Circuits 3, 6, 7, 16

This is the same protocol as the one used to deal with colic in a newborn.

Except for his need for food, the two primary fears of a baby are the fears of being abandoned and being attacked. Therefore, this includes the Panic Protocol given in chapter 4 along with circuit 16 for energizing the colon, as most of the time colic is how a baby expresses her anxiety.

Hatred

See Anger.

Homesickness

See Nostalgia.

Hyperactivity

Circuits 11, 2, (1), 3, 5, 7

Experience has taught me that hyperactivity is a very common sign of anxiety. It is also related to an inadequate coordination between the right and the left hemispheres of the brain, which explains the presence of circuit 11 at the beginning of the protocol.

Hypersomnia (Excessive Daytime Sleepiness)

Circuits 2, 1, 3, (4), (5), (6), 7, (9)

In certain cases, hypersomnia is the solution adopted by a depressed person: sleep is considered the best way to flee the external world where the amount of pain is unbearable. Please refer to the Depression Protocol (chapter 4).

Hypochondria

Circuits 2, 1, 3, 4, 5, 6, 7

This is a constant preoccupation with the functioning of the body and with imagined diseases; hypochondria may become a neurosis when the delusion of ill-health dominates the person's entire life. Circuit 1 against depression can be discontinued as soon as the underlying depressive state passes; continue to do circuits 2, 3, 4 (against negativity, fear, and obsession), and 7 (to restore the fundamental vibration) every day until the phobia of illness is gone.

Impotence

Circuits 2, (1), 3, 4, 5, 9, 19, 21

See also Premature Ejaculation.

Although the reasons for this issue may differ (they are usually related to an ill-managed Oedipus complex or to the fear of functional decline around age 60), fear, obsession, and negativity are constant dominant elements. Apply the same protocol as the one used for premature ejaculation: circuit 2 against negativity, circuit 1 if there is a depressive state, circuit 3 against anxiety, circuit 4 for dealing with obsessions, circuit 5 against hyper-emotionality, circuit 9 to restore the yin/yang balance, circuit 19 to energize the sacral plexus, and circuit 21, which targets the issue more directly.

As a maintenance protocol do circuits 5, 9, 19, and 21.

Inattention, Lack of Concentration, Distraction, Daydreaming

Circuits 11, 5

As far as children are concerned, circuit 11 should be prioritized, because most of the time, there's an inadequate connection between the two hemispheres of the brain. And definitely add circuit 5 against hyper-emotionality.

If dealing with an adult, circuit 1 against depression should be given precedence: escaping the present is a definite way to fight depression. Alternatively, the mind may find itself so hard-pressed that its capacities for attention and memory cannot respond any longer. In that case, use Depression Protocol (chapter 4).

Infections, Repetitive

Circuits (1), 2, 3, 4, 5, (6), 7

Repetitive infections are related to a diminution of the immune system; such a decrease is commonly caused by a deficient, unsatisfying psychological functioning. In most cases, the affected organ reflects an unsolved issue: the bladder, for example, is frequently related to fears and guilt. As mentioned earlier, after her divorce, one of my patients began to be affected by repetitive cystitis from the day she found a new partner; another one had vaginal mycosis for similar reasons.

Some illnesses such as anginas, otitis, or thyroiditis reflect expression issues: the person affected by those problems usually has poor communication skills, keeps emotions and feelings locked inside, and is usually not a very good listener. Many books deal with this symbolism of organs, and to sum up the general idea, let us be reminded of the Tibetan saying: "disease is a letter that our body sends to us." Our body is responsive to what we feel deep down and tells us bluntly what is wrong with us; it does so in its own way without the need for sugar-coated lies.

During the first session, if there's a depressive state caused by the chronic nature of the symptoms, do not hesitate to do circuit 1; add circuit 6 if there's a possibility of a previous traumatic event. Depending on the evolution of the treatment, the circuits may be reduced to circuit 5 (for hyper-emotionality), circuit 7 (for restoring the fundamental vibration), and the circuits more specific to the affected organ.

Insomnia

Circuits 10, 2, 1, 3, 4, 5, 6, 7

Apply circuit 10 because insomnia is often caused by suppressed anger. To that add: circuit 2, as a negative frame of mind is bound to exist; circuit 1 (we previously observed that insomnia could be a symptom of depression); circuit 3, since fear is what makes us stay awake; circuit 4, because obsession has a good chance of emerging; circuit 5, which deals with hyper-emotionality; circuit 6, to clear any "scar" left by a past traumatic incident, which could be the causal event at the source of those sleepless nights; and circuit 7, to restore the fundamental vibration.

The following days, circuits 2, 3, 4, and 7 should be enough.

Inspiration (Lack of)

Circuits 18, 8

As long as the lack of inspiration is not related to an underlying depression, circuit 18 is the circuit to be used when our creativity is blocked. In case of depression, apply the corresponding protocol. As expression and inspiration are closely related, use circuit 8 as well.

Jitters

Circuits 2, 3, 5, 8

See Jitters Protocol, chapter 4.

Letting Go (Inability)

Circuit 4

Circuit 4 is of a paramount importance to help us let go of a problem. When we find ourselves unable to let go, the issue at stake occupies the whole space of our mind; it leaves no room for the expression of our intuition, which is precisely what could provide us with answers.

Libido (Troubles)

Circuits 2, 1, 3, 9, 19, 21

These troubles are commonly related to a depressive state and to anxiety, hence the use of circuits 2, 1, and 3 in the protocol. Circuit 9 restores the yin/yang balance; circuit 19 restores the energy of the sacral plexus, and circuit 21 has a more direct action on the symptoms.

Loss

Circuits 2, 1, 3, 5, 6, 7, (4), (9)

A loss inevitably creates a situation of intense psychological distress. *See* Distress Protocol (chapter 4). Obviously, PBA cannot alter the situation itself; the pain will remain; the sorrow won't disappear magically. But, as already said, someone whose energies have been restored to normal recovers enough to handle the situation in the best possible way considering the circumstances.

Love Sickness

Circuits (10), 2, 1, 3, 4, 5, 6, 7

See also Abandonment, which uses the same protocol. To bring forgiveness, apply circuits 2, 4, 5 (against negativity, obsession, and hyperemotionality), and 7 (restoration of the fundamental vibration). This will be your maintenance treatment.

Lower Back Pain (Lumbago), Severe

Circuits 2, (1), 3, (4), 6, 7, 19

Lower back pain can have different causes, such as osteoarthritis, incorrect posture at the workstation, or even a difference in the length of the lower limbs. In some cases, lower back pain also expresses the existence of total exhaustion and a real difficulty in dealing with current circumstances and pressure, hence the necessity to consider the possibility of depression or obsession.

Severe lumbago, except of course when it is due to bending or lifting something heavy, can indicate suppressed depression, which occurs when you don't want to accept the fact that too much is too much and that you really, really need a break. Your body steps in, so to speak, and warns you that something is wrong with your life. It decides to stop you, and uses the only way it knows, just to make you realize that something definitely has to be changed.

Migraines

Circuits 2, 1, 3, 7, 9

Migraine is very often a psychosomatic reaction due to anxiety or to a vexation, which causes the muscles in the nape of the neck and the upper part of the back to become tense; this severe tension is what induces migraine.

If results are not rapidly obtained, seek professional advice in order to check the state of your vertebrae, as well as of your ophthalmic, sinus, and digestive systems.

Nail-biting (Onychophagia)

Circuits 2, (1), 3, 5, 6, 8

See also Tics and OCD.

The gnawing of nails (on the hands and sometimes the feet) is a major sign of anxiety.

Neck Muscle Tightness (Contractures)

Circuits 2, 1, 3, 6, 7

Intense and prolonged tightness of the neck muscles can be very painful and cause throbbing migraines; it may become chronic and result in severe pains in the trapezius area or in tightness of the jaws.

This condition is related to anxiety and hyper-emotionality. Massages for relaxation, physiotherapy, and osteopathy may succeed in reducing the contractures, but the addition of PBA certainly helps to make those treatments more effective; it also helps to prevent possible relapses.

Nightmares

Circuits 2, 3, 5, 7

Nightmares often correspond to a latent anxiety; stagnant emotional energy can be released in the form of nightmares. When you wake up with your heart racing madly because of a horrible nightmare, remember that all you need is five minutes to do the circuits: this will allow you to go back to sleep peacefully. Do the circuits against negativity, fear, and hyper-emotionality (2, 3, 5). There will be no need to leave your bed if you have learned the circuits by heart or if you have your little notes at your bedside.

Night Terrors

Circuits 3, 6, 7

The application of circuits 3 (against fears), 6 (dealing with scars from a possible past traumatic event), and 7 (restoration of the fundamental vibration) should help a baby or a child to go back to sleep.

Nostalgia, Acute

Circuits 2, 1, 3, 4, 5, 6, 7

Living in the past prevents you from living a full life and recognizing opportunities that come your way.

CASE STUDY
Adapting to a New Environment

An exchange student was depressed and highly emotional; she could not cope with the separation from her home and her family. Being placed in a foreign environment had awakened an old wound (she had been uprooted from her first house at the age of three and made to live elsewhere).

Instead of adapting herself to her circumstances, she decided to acknowledge the fact that the whole experience abroad had been a mistake as well as a total failure. The only thing left to do was to return home.

I started to work on her using the above protocol. She decided to stay and happily made the most of her remaining time in her new environment.

In similar circumstances, do not forget circuit 4 (against obsession), as obsession with the past is something that can linger for a long time.

Obesity

Circuits 2, (1), 3, 4, (5), (6), 9

Priority must be given to circuit 2 because being overweight is definitely responsible for a negative self-image that in turn produces general negativity. Depression may be present; in that case, do circuit 1. Circuit 4 is obviously most necessary, because obsession is what prevents the loss of weight. Think about circuit 6, in case an emotional shock has been the causal element. As a maintenance protocol, do circuits 2, 3, 4, and 9 every morning.

Obsession

Circuits (10), 4, 3, 2, 7, (9)

See Obsession Protocol in chapter 4.

Overwork

Circuits 2, 1

Working in excessive amounts may cause depression; we could compare this special depression to a bone fracture of an athlete who has overestimated his resistance capacity and gone far beyond his limits.

Panic

Circuits 2, 3, (6), 7, (9)

See Panic Protocol, chapter 4.

Perfectionism

Circuits 3, 4

Perfectionism requires circuit 4, as obviously a perfectionist's main issue is not knowing how to let go.

Perfectionism is originally a system of defense used by people who fear criticism and aggressiveness. It has its source in childhood and so has the fear. To keep fear at bay, the unconscious mind basically reasons like this: being perfect is the only way to avoid criticism. It is the only way to stay safe. It is important that you include the Fear Protocol at the beginning of the treatment.

Phobias

Circuits 2, 3, 4, 7

Irrational fear leads to wrong decisions, the consequences of which will negatively impact your life.

Premature Ejaculation

Circuits 2, 1, 3, 4, 5, 9, 19, 21

When we studied circuit 21, we observed that this issue could be experienced as a real nightmare by the affected person and by his partner as well. In some cases, frustrations lead to divorce: the man often refuses the very idea of talking about the issue or simply gets angry when the subject is broached; his sense of self-worth is gone and he feels diminished, believing that there's no cure. He realizes that his partner feels frustrated and this obviously increases his feeling of unease, not to say despair. His partner usually keeps silent about the whole thing and the couple's life is definitely jeopardized.

Premature ejaculation is frequently connected with taboos: it may be related to a feeling of guilt that was the counterpart of the teenager's masturbation habits in the past (the boy had to be quick in case somebody came and discovered the shameful situation; the concept of sin was lurking and somehow persisted in the adult's mind). Another taboo could be the interdiction of incest, which appears when one's partner is idealized to the point that her image and the mother figure become confused and mixed up. Another reason could be the unconscious guilt of adultery that may appear even after a divorce.

In order to try to deal with the situation, start with a thorough rebalancing of the energies: apply circuits 2, 1, 3, 4, and 5 (against negativity, depression, anxiety, obsessions, and hyper-emotionality). Finish with circuit 9 to restore the yin/yang balance. Then, and only then, apply the two circuits that target the issue more specifically: circuit 19 that restores the balance of the sacral plexus and circuit 21 that deals more precisely with sexual difficulties.

On a daily basis, do circuits 5, 9, 19, and 21 until self-confidence returns and noteworthy progress is observed. We usually don't have to wait long for that to happen.

Premenstrual Syndrome

Circuits 2, (1), 5, 9, 19

This well-known syndrome definitely has a negative impact on many young women's lives: the closer they get to the time of their period, the more emotional, miserable, and possibly depressed they feel. These mood shifts of a menstrual cycle are all the more difficult to live with, in that they cannot be controlled by mere willpower: their cause is purely hormonal.

We can remedy this by dealing with negativity (2), and hypersensitivity (5); we also have to restore the yin/yang balance (9) and reenergize the sacral plexus (19). From the twenty-first day of the cycle, be vigilant and do the circuits several times a day if necessary.

Psoriasis

Circuits (1), 3, 2, 12, (4), 5, 6, 7, 13

Psoriasis is a chronic disease, which can be responsible for a painful esthetic prejudice. Its source usually lies in a severe crisis the patient has experienced and has never expressed. Even if the initial crisis is successfully dealt with, at least on the surface, any new experience of pressure will be prone to cause another outbreak. This chronic quality of psoriasis eventually results in biological disorders, with a risk for psoriatic arthritis, which may be very disabling.

Treating the psychosomatic aspect of psoriasis with the help of PBA is highly recommended: first of all, treat the depression that is the direct cause or consequence of psoriasis, then treat the fear that is responsible for the "disconnection" of the ether element.

Oddly, I noticed that circuit 13 (against eczema) was really useful as well (though psoriasis is not a form of eczema). This is why I advise using circuits 12, 5, 7, and 13 as a maintenance protocol.

Psychosomatic Reactions

Circuits 2, (1), 3, 4, 5, 6, 7

An amazingly great number of diseases are psychosomatic reactions to some degree. Going through the entire list is definitely not feasible here. If you suspect such an origin, it will always be good to combine PBA with the classic medical treatment; the effects will certainly be enhanced.

In general, systematically use circuits 2, 3, 4, and 5 (against negativity, fear, obsession, and hyper-emotionality); add circuit 6 (there are certainly "scars" left by the causal event in the energetic system) and 7 (to restore the fundamental vibration). Once again, don't hesitate to do circuit 1 if you think that a depression is looming behind, which is a common occurrence.

To these, add the circuits that correspond to the part of the body you want to treat: circuit 19, if the organs you want to deal with depend on the sacral plexus; circuit 20 if they depend on the solar plexus (notably the digestive sphere, gall bladder, liver, or stomach); circuit 8 if the sinus sphere is concerned; or the specific circuits that correspond to the skin, the bladder, or the colon.

As a maintenance treatment, do circuits 3, 4, and 7 and the specific circuits.

Scalp Diseases

Circuits 12, 2, (1), 3, (4), 5, 6, 7

Diseases affecting the scalp, such as alopecia that occurs without warning, are usually stress-related; most of the time they are the consequence of a shock. Common alopecia, which is progressive, is of hormonal or genetic origin.

Hence the importance of restoring the ether element (circuit 12), and of clearing any "scar" that could have been left by ancient trauma (circuit 6), as well as of combating fear (circuit 3), negativity (circuit 2), and sometimes depression (circuit 1).

As a maintenance protocol, keep doing circuit 12, circuit 3, and circuit 7 for a long time. A few weeks are required to appreciate the results of this protocol, which is really effective in most cases.

Self-deprecation

Circuits 2, 1. 3, (4), (5), (6), 7, (9)

See also Depression.

Once someone starts losing her sense of self-worth and once this self-deprecating attitude begins to show systematically (especially if this type of behavior did not exist before), then, you may be sure that depression is close. There's no need to wait, just apply the Depression Protocol.

Spasmophilia

Circuits 2, 1, 3, 6, 7

Spasmophilia is a disabling disorder that takes different forms in different people. Its most common aspect is a generalized state of involuntary muscular contraction, accompanied by a state of profound anxiety and a tingling sensation, notably in the hands and feet. Other symptoms include involuntary movements of the eyes, kidney pains, colitis, severe cramps, or a depressive state induced by the change of seasons.

PBA may be very helpful in these cases; a cure of trace elements is also recommended.

Stammering

Circuits 2, (1), 3, 5, 6, 8

See also Tics and OCD.

Stammering may be considered a form of tic.

Stomach Ulcers

Circuits (10), 2, 3, 5, (6), 7, 20

Stomach ulcers are another psychosomatic condition, and not the least one.

Apply circuits 2 and 3 (against negativity and fear), circuit 5 (against hyper-emotionality), circuit 6 (if the causal event has been traumatic), and 20 (to energize the solar plexus); this last circuit feeds energy to the stomach. Don't forget circuit 10 (to deal with suppressed anger) if the ulcer is related to an unsolved conflict or to a bullying incident.

Stress (Temporary)

Circuits 3, 7

Stress can have an impact on all aspects of your existence. It must be managed before it escalates.

Tics and OCD
(Obsessive Compulsive Disorders)

Circuits 2, (1), 3, 5, 6, 8

Tics are definitely stress related (constant flicker of the eyelids for example); so are obsessive compulsive disorders (such as repetitive washing of hands caused by fear of contamination). Tics are successfully treated with circuit 3 against fear and possibly circuit 1 if you suspect a depressive state; circuit 5 against hyper-emotionality and 6 to remove the scars left by previous trauma improve the situation remarkably: the children I have treated this way have recovered in a short time.

I always recommend that the parents "let go" of the problem instead of focusing on it, which only worsens the situation. Pressure definitely won't help and anxiety will just build faster; all that will be achieved will be an exacerbation of the child's anxiety and tics. The first thing to do is to seem to notice nothing.

Nonetheless we have to remember that tics are warning signals: as soon as they reappear, we may safely say that another incident has destabilized the child again; parents are familiar with this pattern and have often told me: "something must have happened at school; he has started to stammer again."

Tonsillitis, Repetitive

Circuits 2, (1), 3, (4), 5, (6), 7, 8

See also Infections, Repetitive.

Expression is definitely an issue here; unsaid words and unexpressed feelings generate a serious disturbance. To start with, apply circuit 1 if depression is present, circuit 4 in case of obsession, and circuit 6 if the presence of a previous trauma is detected. As a maintenance protocol, apply circuit 5 against hyper-emotionality and circuit 8 to enhance expression on a regular basis.

Trichotillomania
(Compulsive Hair Pulling)

Circuits 2, (1), 3, 5, 6, 8

See also Tics and OCD.

This is a pathologically powerful urge that causes someone to pull out her own hair constantly. As this is a compulsive disorder, please refer to the section that deals with OCD.

Uprooting

Circuits 2, 1, 3, 7, 19

Uprooting can be expressed by a loss of reference marks. It may resonate with an earlier psychological suffering, such as when we had to adapt to new circumstances during our childhood: perhaps we had to move to another city or country and lost the familiar company of our friends or grandparents; perhaps our parents divorced or we had to adapt to a new school.

Whatever the reason behind the loss of our original way of life, it will remain ingrained in us; then, in our future life, whenever we are confronted by something new (a new job, a new house), we will unconsciously be reminded of that first time when we had been deprived of our familiar surroundings.

Depression may occur and perhaps seem the more mysterious when we consciously want the very change that is making us sick. The inner conflict of course creates imbalance. At some level, handling change is perceived as scary and clinging to the comfort zone seems more tempting, even when wanting to experience something new is also there.

But things can get more complicated: the fear of losing one's familiar environment may express itself by a fear of putting down roots. This is not as paradoxical as it looks: as long as you have no deep roots, you don't risk losing them. This explains certain behaviors of chronic instability and fear of commitment (personal, professional, or geographical): more often than not, people affected by this predicament share the same story: they lost their familiar surroundings at an early age and their unconscious mind has decided to never allow the painful experience to recur.

The perspective of losing everything that is or has become familiar may generate a real panic with certain fragile persons: I saw quite a number of women who had followed their Army husbands overseas succumb to depression when the time came for them to pack and go back home. Logically, they should have been happy to see their families and their home country again; after all, for months and months, they had talked about this reunion with their family with great anticipation, only to find when the moment came, that they could not handle the depressing idea of leaving their adopted new home.

Whether we deal with a child who has lost his whereabouts because he has been sent to summer camp without having been asked in the first place, or with an adult who cannot cope with an old painful experience recurring, we have to take into account the factors of fear and depression. There may be somatic repercussions at the level of the sacral plexus (or root chakra) such as kidney problems, sciatica, fibromas (nonmalignant tumors of the connective tissue), or a prostate problem; this is why we have to remember to restore the energetic balance at the level of the sacral plexus (circuit 19).

Vaginal Mycosis, Repetitive

Circuits 2, 3, 4, 5, 7, 19

See also Infections, Repetitive.

Work on guilt.

6

Five Golden Rules for Retaining Energy Balance

Being careful about the balance of our energies is just one aspect of how we can care for ourselves and others; we also need to retain our energies once their balance has been properly restored.

Having understood that thought *is* energy and that this energy produces the largest part of the vital force that animates us, we have to find a way to control the way our thoughts drift toward negativity and deplete our supply of energy. We have to break the patterns responsible for our addiction to negativity. If we can't do this, then we will lose what we gained from restoring our energy; we will find ourselves in the position of somebody trying to fill a colander. It definitely takes a conscious choice to disengage from the old patterns and to optimize the way we live.

In order to avoid negative thought and behavior patterns, we have to acknowledge and respect certain rules that I call "the five golden rules." They will look familiar to you, of course, as I did not invent them. However, I want you to awaken something in you that you may have forgotten and that can assist you in changing the way you approach things.

These rules are:

1. Avoid unnecessary stress.
2. Avoid dwelling on the same old stories.
3. Avoid guilt (make the distinction between fault and mistake).
4. Protect yourself against external negativity.
5. Live in the Now.

Rule Number 1

Avoid Unnecessary Stress

I'm sure you have noticed that your perception of an event is often more consequential than the event itself. Anxiety just increases the significance of an incident, which, on the other hand, is experienced as non-meaningful or as less traumatic if you are relaxed at the time it happens.

Learning how to keep things in perspective helps us to make a less emotional evaluation of the situation and prevents us from becoming overwhelmed by a minor event (this is called "relativization"). You may have your own recipe to help you to consider things in context. If not, you are welcome to have mine: my little technique may seem simple, still it helps me to save half my energy. As soon as something unpleasant happens to me, the first thing I do is to ask myself: "Am I going to think about it in five years' time?" If the answer is negative, as it is most of the time, I reject the incident as non-significant. This does not mean that I won't try my best to find a solution, because I will, but in the process I'll feel more relaxed and save valuable energy within my solar plexus.

Let me give an example: imagine I have to catch a plane and have a flat tire on my way to the airport. Now, I have two options: either I lose control of my nerves and work myself into such a state of angered and flustered frustration that I lose all my energy with the result that I eventually miss my plane. Or I just calmly ask myself the following question: "Am I going to think about this in five years [here I plug in the specific date,* five years in the future]?" When it seems clear that I will not, then the incident does not warrant my losing my precious energy on it.

Having stepped aside from my situation for a minute, I let go of the negative emotions and recover my composure and inner calm; because of this relaxed state of mind, I am open to opportunities and I am in a position to spot a friend who happens to drive along the road and is happy to help me out. Other possibilities are allowed to emerge when we do not give in to negativity. Instead of letting anger dominate our thoughts, or transmitting a signal to the universe that we expect nothing good, we can tap into the knowledge that, somehow, things will be pulled together in order to assist us.

This approach is pertinent regarding all the little things that continually upset us; just take a minute to think about the dozens of incidents that have been a cause of tension to you since the beginning of this current month: arriving late at a movie, a distasteful remark from a colleague, the "bad" school results of your son, the traffic at peak hours. Dozens of mini events ate up your energy and were absolutely not worth it. Our objective here is to find ways to save as much of our energy as we can. We have to let the emotional charge of the incident dissipate by stepping away from the scene.

This is how you embrace the first rule: "I refuse to lose my energy because of an incident that I will have forgotten in five years' time. Putting this event into context and seeing it for what it really is, gives me the quietness of mind necessary to find solutions for it."

Rule Number 2

Avoid Dwelling on the Same Old Stories

Now what do we do about those things that *will* still occupy our mind five years from now? Rule number two tells us to avoid brooding end-

---

*I suggest making the small effort to state the precise date, because our brain won't react if we are too vague ("in five years time"). A sentence that becomes automatic won't alert the brain; things have to be said and done in full awareness in order to put the brain on alert.

lessly over the same past event: the more anxiety or anger we project on an issue, the bigger it will get. A brooding attitude definitely won't help; only in letting go, accepting, and getting some distance from the incident will a solution be found. New insights will be triggered when tension is released.

A most common example is the case of a young couple obsessed with the desire to have a baby. Nothing seems to be wrong with them; fertility tests have come back clear, and yet, no pregnancy seems possible. After a few years and a lot of misery, the decision to adopt is finally made. Two months after the adoption, the long-awaited pregnancy occurs.

Similar are cases of persons who are obsessed with their weight and for whom the most severe slimming diets never seem to work. Oddly enough, something different happens when, during a summer holiday, they allow themselves to relax, forget about their weight issues, and enjoy their food. On the way back home, they can't help feeling a bit nervous: what are the scales going to say? Somehow the scales are quite happy: unexpectedly much weight has been shed. Holiday has been a time of relaxation and the weight problem has just been set aside.

Some of us may have experienced a sudden loss of memory during an assignment at school: what was that famous general's name again? We try so hard to remember that no name at all pops into our mind, not until we go back home and have let go of all the strain and the tension. This is why teachers often suggest to students who are taking a test not to waste time on a question that eludes them, but to go back to it only after the whole test has been completed. Pressure obviously does not help in such circumstances.

Incidents such as the following may also have occurred to some of us: we meet with a friend who excitedly tells us something like: "As soon as I stopped worrying about meeting someone, I met the love of my life." What happens is that we are so fixated on an issue that nothing else is allowed to enter our mind; the question that worries us takes the whole space and leaves room for nothing else. Our memory, our intuition, and the messages from our unconscious mind are gagged or blocked out because a single question invades the whole space of our mind, denying us access to a larger perspective. Obviously no answer can be found this way. We have to let go.

To recap: when facing a problem, ask yourself whether it still will be a concern of yours in five years' time: if the answer is negative, gain a fresh perspective, give the situation its real worth, and do not allow yourself to repeatedly relive it in your head. If the answer is positive, try not to obsess and, if after some reasonable time, you realize that you are still not moving on, and that the problem is still there, then you have to decide consciously to let it go, even if for a limited duration (a few hours or a few days). Otherwise the solution will evade you forever.

If you make the conscious effort to put the problem aside before going to sleep, then your intuition will have a chance to present you with an answer (a kind of "flash") the minute you wake up. Or a dream (that will perhaps have to be decoded) will send you a message from your unconscious mind. You will find yourself connected to a field of possibilities that goes far beyond the limited access you have when you go around and around on the same thought. A sleepless night will clearly be of no assistance at all either. You have to break free of the mental drama.

Following the second rule means that you do your best to avoid obsession with an issue, however serious it appears, and you decide not to dwell on the same old miseries, knowing that doing so will only bring bitterness and exhaustion; it will just corrode your energy.

Rule Number 3

Avoid Guilt
(Distinguish between Fault and Mistake)

Our system of education is largely based upon guilt. Something along the way has gone wrong and the two separate notions of responsibility and guilt have become mixed up. Throughout history, this deliberate confusion has allowed certain people or institutions to gain power over others.

In reality, when we find ourselves attuned to our inner sense of personal accountability and duty, then we connect to a positive energy that is uplifting; on the other hand, if we allow guilt to get the best of us, whatever the situation, we become attached to a negative energy.

"Fault" and "mistake" are very different concepts, yet the two are often mixed up. Saying "It's your fault" is not the same as saying "You've made a mistake." In the second case, you did not willingly plan to do something bad or wrong. There was no deliberate intention of doing something bad or harming someone.

Imagine a young woman who is eager to look pretty for her fiancé and takes a little too much time with her make-up; the couple misses the booking at the fancy restaurant and the young man accuses the young lady "It's your fault!" Is it? Obviously not, as the young woman is not guilty of any "bad" intention; she did not plan to be late. She is just responsible for not having scheduled the appropriate time for her make-up.

Nevertheless, such seemingly minor incidents do produce a subliminal guilt within us. Therefore, before experiencing those poisonous whirls of guilt and downward spiral, ask yourself: "Did I honestly do this on purpose?" If the answer is negative, then just reject the guilt. Unnecessary guilt will just drain you; it certainly is not a helpful energetic choice.

This does not mean that you don't try to fix the problem, but that you do so without the weight of guilt on your shoulders. Most of us do tend to feel blameworthy all the time and listen to the nagging inner voice that systematically condemns us no matter what. Then, for example, if our children happen to have learning difficulties or psychological issues, the first thought that comes to mind is "Where did I go wrong?" and that spontaneous thought is immediately followed by a feeling of intense guilt. We usually deny ourselves the right to make a simple mistake as though we were supposed to be all-knowing in parental matters.

Mistakes, however, are part of our human condition and are there to teach us. They are part of our apprenticeship, and they seem to be the only way at our disposal to acquire experience. As Neale Donald Walsch put it in his *Conversations with God,* "One can realize who one really is only in realizing who one is not."

Clearly, we have to be responsible and do our best to fix whatever problem has been created by our lack of attention or our distraction. But taking responsibility and not blaming others signifies staying positive, whereas feeling guilty for no reason diminishes or even negates the action that is supposed to fix things.

It is good to rediscover that spirit that used to animate us when we were children: "I did not do it on purpose!" cried little four-year-old you after having broken your mom's favorite cup. At that age, you were still intuitively aware of the difference between mistake and fault.

Rule Number 4

Protect Yourself Against External Negativity

Any miserable or aggressive person charges us with negative energies.

We have all had the experience of coming across a friend who, for a full hour, describes his miserable life to us, only to part with us with a broad smile, saying: "I feel *so* much better now!" But *you* obviously don't. You feel dejected and drained all of a sudden as if you had soaked up your friend's negativity. And you have. An aggressive person may load you with negativity in the same way. This process has been described with accuracy in the popular book *Celestine Prophecy* (by James Redfield). We inhabit a world of vampires, even if they are unconscious vampires, and many of us are endlessly feeding on other people's energies. This is why moral harassment is so common: an energy-sucking bully feeds on his victim's fear or submission; hence the vital necessity to protect our own energy system and make it strong.

To do so, we can build a specific energy, which will serve as a shield between us and external negativity. This is certainly feasible: let's keep in mind again that thought is energetic in nature and that we do have a say in transforming our energetic output. We choose the kind of energy we want. This choice is dependent on the content of our thoughts. The comparison between a brain and a computer seems perfectly appropriate in this particular case. But this comparison serves only the purpose of clarification: obviously, as long as we do not ask for anything, our brain will stay put. In the same manner, there are lots of programs on a hard disk but as long as you do not click on the disk, the programs don't show up.

So, let us decide to take deliberate action in order to protect our energies and let us ask our brain to build an energy shield for us. Here is how to proceed:

+ Define what kind of program you want.
+ Give a name to this program (you need an icon to represent it).
+ Learn how to make it work (click on the icon).

Define the Program

We want an energy that protects us; we don't want an energy that makes us indifferent to the world. (If a friend needs our help, we are not going to reject him with the excuse that our energetic system finds itself at risk with him. On the other hand it is clearly not necessary that we let ourselves get contaminated by his misery.)

We may compare this concept of an energy that protects us and at the same time allows us to help with a fireman's suit: a fireman who enters a burning house without his suit may become a hero but his bravery has a strong chance of being ineffective, whereas putting on his suit protects him and allows him to do his job the best he can.

Give a Name to the Program

You can readily give it any name of your choosing, as this process is only a convention between your mind and yourself. "Shield," "screen," or anything you choose is just fine. Just stick to the name once it has been selected. Remember, a program responds to one name only. I have called mine "neutral shield" because we obviously need a shield as a protection between the world and us; it's neutral too, because the acupressure circuits we use on ourselves produce a positive energy, whereas the energy we want to protect ourselves against is negative. But then, any name will do.

How to Click

It's simple: any time you find yourself in the company of a very unhappy or aggressive person, don't wait, breathe in deeply, then hold your breath for a moment. This is needed, since if you try to build up your energy of protection in a distracted way, you will not create a situation in which your brain is clearly informed that something is happening. However, holding your breath for a few seconds makes your brain quickly realize that something is wrong and helps it to become instantly alert.

Once you are aware and no longer distracted, just say clearly in your head the special name you have chosen ("neutral shield" for example). This is all you have to do, as the energy of protection sets itself automatically.

Likewise, when you are on the phone and find that the person you are talking to is very hostile or aggressive, just find a quick excuse to make the person hold on for a few seconds: breathe in, hold, give the order to your brain, and calmly listen to what the person has to say.

Naturally, you will not become indifferent, a mean word will still hurt and you will still shed tears if a friend's story is really too sad. But once the situation is over, you will not be destabilized; you will have avoided absorbing all the negativity as well as the mental exhaustion. Your energy will remain intact. I have yet to be told that this does not work.

In my daily practice, I used to spend the whole day in the company of depressed people who were often going through heartbreaking situations. I would never have been able to cope without that energy of protection, which helped me to help without weighing me down with intense negativity, All those years were extremely emotionally intense and I really had to protect myself the best I could. Yet, truly, none of my patients' problems ever left me indifferent. I was touched by their stories. But I did not absorb their negativity and this is exactly what I recommend to anyone who has direct contact with people's energies during their day at work (massage therapists, osteopaths, medical staff, beauticians, hairdressers, and so forth): "Think of creating your energy of protection as often as possible. Do not let yourself become a sponge for the misery of the world." I also apply this myself sometimes when watching the news on TV.

Live in the Now

It is common knowledge nowadays that we receive cosmic energy as well as telluric energy when we are in our space-time continuum. However, when we disconnect ourselves and are *not* in our own space-time continuum, we deprive ourselves of a major source of energy. Our space-time continuum is by definition the present time; we disconnect ourselves whenever we are living in the past or in the future or bouncing from the past to the future. Then we are no longer living in the Now, which is our specific time frame. Then we are no longer attuned to the vibrations of the time frame where we belong.

Living in the Past

Among other things, the past often signifies resentment, sadness, nostalgia, remorse, anger, or grudge. Let's talk about anger for a minute: certain religious systems teach us the importance of forgiveness, which is presented to us as a spiritual act, and I respect that. Nevertheless, we could also interpret things a bit differently: to forgive is to let go, to let the past be the past and to give priority to the present; it signifies a readjustment to the energies of the present. This is quantum reality.

It is wonderful to witness the reconciliation of spiritual teachings with the latest discoveries in physics, which is happening more and more. I realize that it is hard sometimes to leave behind our regrets, anger, or resentment, but in so doing we do keep our energies safe and sound. This is all the more necessary in that living in the past won't alter things an iota.

Living in the Future

Many of us dream up situations that *could* happen, only to discover later that these scenarios did not correspond to what was in store for us. Our negative mental dialogues imagine situations, which create a scary and anxiety-filled universe: this is how our energetic system becomes depleted.

Our mind produces the worst scenarios and gloomy projections into the future; we almost never imagine that we have won the lottery and that our family is healthy and happy. We envision disasters with horrific chain-reactions. A member of our family is late for dinner, which prompts us into thinking "accident" instead of "happy meeting with an old acquaintance." "What-if" is a bad adviser, which wears us down.

I remember one of my patients who had heard a rumor about his employer firing people. As he had been the last person to be hired, he started to imagine the worst: he began to obsess about having to pay for his house without a salary and that he would not be able to spare money for the education fees for his children. Soon he was on antidepressant drugs. After six months, no one in his firm had been fired. My patient had wasted all his precious energy imagining things that were not going to happen, and had suffered from depression for just an illusion.

I have very often dealt with young undergraduate students who were anxiety-ridden because they had lost their grip on the current reality and were endlessly reviewing scenarios involving their failure, the reaction of their disappointed parents, and their prospects or rather lack of prospects for the year following their failure. Their negative imagination deprived them of all willpower and grounded sense of purpose. Besides applying five point touch therapy to help them to recover, I usually said something like the following: "Failure is to be taken into consideration the day you have your results. Just holding the thought of a possible failure drags you down and prevents you from studying. Anticipating failure can only limit your much-needed energy. Instead of channeling it into a disastrous storyline, you could just concentrate on the present."

A Problem Has to Be Dealt with the Day it Occurs

I don't agree with the mind-set that says to be prepared for the worst means to imagine the worst beforehand. What if the worst does not happen? It is absolutely of no use whatsoever to imagine different possible versions of mishaps, which may or more probably may never happen. In other words, we have to deal with our reality in the Now. We have to avoid a split, which induces only fatigue, and which occurs when we are physically in one place and mentally in another reality. We have to live in our specific time frame. This is our field of action.

Yes, the future has to be taken into account and projects and plans have to be made; nevertheless once these plans have been decided upon, it is necessary to return to the present time and to be watchful for any synchronous events that might present themselves to help us with whatever we need to achieve.

Thought is a powerful creative process, so creative that if we could really trust ourselves completely, we could experience events almost automatically responding to our wishes. We could influence outcomes by directing our energy into the probability we want to be materialized. In the world of quantum physics, thought is what connects us to the field of probabilities. This is far from being the case for most of us who doubt the workings of the field and consider separation instead of interconnectedness. Negativity is a potent polluting agent.

To sum up, the fifth rule is to live in the Now in order to best absorb and benefit from the specific telluric and cosmic energies of our time frame.

These five rules have to be kept in mind if we want to retain our energy; discipline is needed, but it is a small price to pay if we are to enjoy the balance of our energies that has been restored by the PBA circuits.

Conclusion

There are two ways to live one's life: one is to think that miracles
do not exist; the other is to think that everything is a miracle.

ALBERT EINSTEIN

Don't feel intimidated by the apparent complexity of the protocols I
have introduced here. They really are easily done once you have become
familiar with the 22 circuits (especially the ten most commonly used
ones introduced in chapter 2).

Over the years, my daily experience as a therapist has demonstrated
that tensions start to dissolve and that any weight on the chest disappears at an early stage of a session. Patients and participants in my workshops all confirm this. A state of relief and deep relaxation is induced
in a short time: a couple of minutes are often what it takes for the person to feel much better, and this happens long before the session ends.
Nonetheless, you have to be firm in your determination and finish the
work thoroughly, without skipping anything.

If you are working on yourself, even if you feel much better, be adamant
and keep doing the protocols several times on the first day and once a day
as a maintenance treatment until you feel sure that the issue is really gone.

I also want to remind you that PBA is a preventive treatment as well;
don't wait until something has gone seriously wrong. We human beings
tend to resign ourselves to some kind of natural lethargy and act or react

only once a problem arises. Furthermore, many of us have a natural disposition to negativity, which is exactly the factor that prevents us from working on ourselves. I therefore recommend that you do at least circuits 2, 3, and 7 every morning when you get up. This will take only a couple of minutes of your time, which is really not much to ask, and the effects on your day will be amazing. Even if you feel great and if you think that everything is fine with your life, just devote a couple of minutes to those circuits.

The participants at my workshops are usually in a great shape for weeks afterward. However, a few of them occasionally come to consult me a few weeks after and I find that, once again, they are in a negative state. To the question "Have you done your circuits?" the answer is invariably "No." They say: "Well at the beginning, I did. But then, I felt so great that I just forgot about them."

Negativity seems to be another kind of gravitational force: just as gravity made an apple fall on Newton's head (so legend says), negativity tries to drag us down and prevent us from staying positive. Once again, let's keep in mind that the more positive we are, the more resilient and strong our energetic system is; we have the possibility to hold its full capacity and increase our vitality.

To remain positive definitely requires a conscious effort; we need to take responsibility for our own lives and successfully deal with any misfortune that comes our way. As soon as we stop being vigilant, the "gravity" force of negativity pulls us down. When we are "down," our mental clarity is blurred and our energy flow is constricted. The more unwell we feel, the more indolent we are, and the less we feel like reacting and doing something to get better.

I find that the image of the race between the eagle and the turtle in La Fontaine's well-known seventeenth century poem is symbolic of this situation. Poor turtle desperately tries to walk as fast as it can to reach its goal; it finds countless obstacles along its way and is unable to foresee any of them as they materialize at the last minute. Meanwhile the eagle quietly flies straight to its goal because of its high altitude position. When we are in a positive frame of mind, we are a bit like an eagle, only to become turtles again as soon as negativity gets the best of us. As this book has shown, psycho-bio-acupressure is a really extraordinary tool that requires only some minutes to control most of our destructive emotions, but apathy has to be overcome, again and again, for us to exert our willpower and do our circuits regularly. As for myself, I do circuits 2, 3, and 7 every morning. After that, I briefly analyze the events of the previous day and focus on what I may expect on this new day. If I feel a little depressed, I do circuit 1; if I sense hyper-emotionality, I do circuit 5; in case a problem takes too much space in my mind, I do circuit 4. The whole thing has become a routine process. Very often, when having a difficult time, and when I don't feel like doing the circuits, I nevertheless will myself to do them; ten minutes later, I'm rewarded, because I feel so much better and ready to start a new and very busy day.

Don't hesitate to begin a similar routine: you'll rapidly observe that you feel more dynamic and more capable of facing the challenges that come your way. Of course, your circumstances won't have changed and your life will basically be the same, but your personal perspective will be different and you will definitely feel stronger and able to cope with whatever it is you have to experience. This is what I wanted to share with you; I wanted to give you the means to handle things thanks to five acupressure points.

I would like now to insist on two notions that I consider crucial and that may encourage you to make five point touch therapy a daily routine. They illustrate the concept that our reality is directly related to our thoughts and the choices we make.

First, the image we have of ourselves is decisive. It literally compels us to act according to it, hence the importance of improving it. A distorted or negative perception of reality may create a downward spiral for us. A negative thought should be immediately followed by a positive thought. Saying to yourself, "I'm old and tired, I expect nothing more from my life," can beneficially be replaced with "My body is still strong and I still have time to do things in my life." Instead of thinking, "I'm fat and no one is going to love me ever," try to say: "I will find solutions to all these problems that are responsible for my extra weight."

Our health is the mirror of our thoughts and emotions; our attitudes about life determine our amount of vital energy and definitely impact causality. PBA allows us to hold a positive state of mind that will help us build a positive image of ourselves.

The second notion that is extremely important to keep in mind is that *it is our duty (toward ourselves and toward other people) to stay attuned to positive energies as much as we can.* This is clearly a duty that we owe to ourselves, since we clearly depend on our body and our organs to stay in good health; we've seen that our energetic system is highly responsive to the content of our thoughts and that the best way to maintain a good balance is to provide it with the best energy available.

This is a duty toward other people as well, as we are all part of the one universal field. The farther we travel on our way to positivity, the more we radiate, the more we are able to bring along those around us. Our interconnectedness will in the end bring about new patterns for everyone. Once again, this is quantum reality. It is as simple as that.

Allow me an anecdote here: at the time of the 9/11 disaster, I had my practice in New Caledonia. Due to the time difference between there and the East coast of the United States it was nighttime for us when the planes hit the towers, and we were not aware of the events occurring in New York.

I was stunned the next day when most of my patients reported to me that they had not slept at all or extremely badly the night before. My daughter who was nine at that time had been very sick that night without any medical reason. The enormous energy of terror and panic, which had swept the whole world, had hit New Caledonia as well in spite of our blessed unawareness of the attack. That immense energy created by millions of negative thoughts all over the earth had altered the energetic state of the world so that even during their sleep (or lack of sleep) people in New Caledonia had been able to perceive the huge wave of fear and terror that had swept over the planet.

This event demonstrated even more to me how tightly interdependent all humans are; it showed how an event that is heavily emotionally charged, which directly affects a limited part of the planet, can affect the rest of the world. Apparently, global disasters make interconnectedness tangible in a way we are not generally aware of. Keeping in mind the staggering implications of this connection helps us all and allows us to live richer lives.

In this light, let me stress again the paramount importance of staying attuned to positive energies as much as possible; this is our responsibility and this can be done through the daily use of the five point PBA circuits.

The Evolution of Five Point Touch Therapy

I was told once that five point acupuncture was as ancient a healing art as traditional acupuncture, but that it was reserved for a handful of initiates (possibly because it involves a higher vibration level).

As for me, this is not what attracted me in the first place.

During a workshop in which I enrolled in 1988, I was told that this particular form of acupuncture existed in Australia. However, it was at a short workshop in 1992 that I was introduced to what was called at the time "energetic medicine." We were required to study the first book written by Doctor Patrick Véret—*La médecine cosmogénétique ou l'Energo-médecine* (Cosmogenetic Medicine or Energetic Medicine)— along with another of his books, *La spasmophilie enfin vaincue* (Conquering Spasmophilia).* Some circuits introduced in this book, particularly the one against negativity and the one that restores the ether element, were brought to my knowledge through those readings.

Since that time, I have explored much further and discovered other circuits through a lengthy correspondence with Doctor Patrick

---

*Doctor Véret did not limit his research to this special form of five point acupuncture; his work also involved trace elements and essential amino acids as well, in what he called Nutripuncture. (See *Nutripuncture: Stimulating the Energy Pathways of the Body Without Needles* [Rochester, Vt.: Healing Arts Press, 2012].)

Jouhaud, a doctor from Limoges, France, who works with energies as well. As far as I am aware, more than 300 circuits exist, which deal with different issues such as asthma, sciatica, hypertension, sinus conditions, and so forth.

I decided to select some of those circuits that I found had much more impact on negative psychological states of mind than on their intended physical targets. For example, I ascertained that the circuit associated with clearing the energetic impact of *physical* trauma has in fact a far greater effect on *psychological* issues. In the same way, circuit 7 for the restoration of the fundamental vibration in all energetic centers is *the* perfect circuit to break down all conditioning patterns inherited from childhood.

Over time, I selected and modified a certain number of circuits; others I discovered, and eventually I found myself working with the twenty-two circuits introduced in this book. As for the notion of triggering five points simultaneously, other researchers whose genius I fully acknowledge have intuited the concept. As I worked with the circuits, I noticed that the efficacy of the circuits improved when a specific sequence was respected: this is how I decided to group them into definite protocols, each protocol corresponding to a special negative state.

Then, as already mentioned, I resolved to change from acupuncture to acupressure, first using patches before deciding to use manual pressure. A major, albeit apparently paradoxical, benefit of acupressure is that it has quicker and more effective results than the triggering of pressure points with needles. It can be applied on the spot in emergency situations. The other benefit of acupressure is that it is a self-help technique.

The techniques I have shared with you in this book are based upon this progressive evolution: the selection of certain acupuncture circuits, as well as the discovery of radically different applications for them, grouping them into protocols, my long clinical observation and experience, and the affirming experience of sharing all this in many workshops.

About the Author

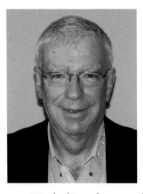

My father, Doctor Pierre-Noël Delatte passed away unexpectedly on the 5th of August 2012. He had dedicated the past 20 years of his life to developing and sharing a technique that helped thousands of people around the world. His biggest desire and mission on this Earth was to help people. He loved humanity and spent his life improving the lives of as many individuals as possible.

He believed strongly in preventive health care rather than curative methods and this led to the development of psycho-bio-acupressure (PBA). Through PBA he was able to help many people liberate themselves from the negative impacts of traumatic experiences. He dreamed of a world with enough PBA practitioners and educators so that everyone would have access to this healing method.

He lived his life with great faith and humanity in everything that he did. He has left a great legacy on this Earth and will continue to help people through his books and the excellent team that he formed at the Delatte Institute of Psycho-Bio-Acupressure.

We loved him and thank him for creating and sharing this wonderful method and new way of life.

ALEXANDRE DELATTE

Resources

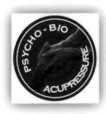 The Delatte Institute of Psycho-Bio-Acupressure (Institut Delatte de Psycho-Bio-Acupressure) was created to spread PBA around the world as well as to protect and support its practitioners. The objectives of the institute are to

+ Organize workshops all around the world, teaching people how to use psycho-bio-acupressure.
+ Train practitioners and teachers and deliver the relevant diplomas.
+ Federate and protect PBA professionals.
+ Establish relationships between PBA professionals and clients.
+ Create initiatives that will allow the development and evolution of PBA.

It is therefore through this institute that all workshops will be organized.

There are five levels of PBA workshops. Levels 1 and 2 are available to anyone who wishes to gain a further understanding of PBA and to be educated by an accredited teacher. Levels 3, 4, and 5 are reserved for people who want to use PBA professionally. To check for workshops or practitioners in your area, please visit **www.psycho-bio-acupressure .com**. If no workshops are scheduled in your area, please contact the institute directly at **contact@institut-delatte.org** about organizing one.

Index

Page numbers in *italics* refer to illustrations.

abandonment, 152–53

accessibility, 5

accidents, 153

acne, 91–95, *91–95*

acupuncture points, 13

allergies, 81–84, *82–84*

anger, 70–74, *71–74*, 154

anguish, 154

anorexia, 27, 154

anxiety, 37–41, *38–41*, 154–55

apathy, 27, 155

application of technique, 21–22

asthma, 81–84, *82–84*, 155–56

attention deficit disorder, 76–80, *77–80*

auras, 13

baby, desire to have, 159, 181

back pain, 166

batteries, 22

bedwetting, 96–97, 156

beliefs, 133–34

bladder, 96–100, *97–100*

brain, 14–15, 76–80, *77–80*

bulimia, 27, 156

bullying, 139, 156

Callahan, Roger, 23

case studies

   adapting to a new environment, 168

   after an accident, 153

   attention deficit disorder, 76–77

   coping with bullying, 139

   cystitis, 96

   eczema, 86

   family separation, 9–10

   fear of driving test, 8–9

   grief, 7

   infant panic, 10–12

   numbness after a shock, 137–38

   obsessions, 144–45

   obsessive fear, 141–42

   panic attacks, 143

public speaking, 145–46
use of symbolic objects, 105–6
chakras, 13
chemical challenges, 26
Chopra, Deepak, 134
chronic fatigue, 157
circuit 1, 27–31, *28–31*, 135–38
circuit 2, 32–36, *33–36*, 135–38,
191–92
circuit 3, 37–41, *38–41*, 135–38,
191–92
circuit 4, 42–45, *42–45*, 135–38
circuit 5, 46–50, *47–50*
circuit 6, 51–55, *52–55*, 135–38
circuit 7, 56–59, *56–59*, 135–38
circuit 8, 60–64, *61–64*
circuit 9, 65–69, *66–69*
circuit 10, 70–74, *71–74*, 135–38
circuit 11, 76–80, *77–80*
circuit 12, 81–84, *82–84*
circuit 13, 85–90, *87–90*
circuit 14, 91–95, *91–95*
circuit 15, 96–100, *97–100*
circuit 16, 101–4, *101–4*
circuit 17, 105–10, *107–10*
circuit 18, 111–14, *111–14*
circuit 19, 115–19, *116–19*
circuit 20, 120–24, *121–24*
circuit 21, 125–28, *126–28*
circuit 22, 129–32, *129–32*
colic, 157
colon, 101–4, *101–4*, 158
Conception Vessel 4, 42, *42*, 112, *112*
Conception Vessel 5, 129, *129*
Conception Vessel 17, 30, *30*, 39, *39*
Conception Vessel 24, 77, *77*

conflicts, 158
creativity, 111–14, *111–14*
cystitis, 96–100, *97–100*, 158, 164

dairy products, 85
daydreaming, 163
depression, 21–22, *22*, 27–31, *28–31*,
159, 176–77
Depression Protocol, 9–10, 138–41
distal, 20
Distress Protocol, 7, 135–38, 153
divorce. *See* abandonment
Dogna, Michel, 23
dorsal, 20
doubt, 32
driving test, 8–9
dyslexia, 76–80, *77–80*, 159–60

ear infections, 160
eczema, 85–90, *87–90*, 160–61
Elmiger, Jean, 23, 140
ether element, 81–84, *82–84*
exam jitters, 161
exhaustion, 27
expression, enhancing, 60–64,
61–64

family separation, 9–10
fear, 37–41, *38–41*, 141–43, 161
fear of driving test, 8–9
fifth golden rule, 187–89
first golden rule, 179–80
five elements, 81
five golden rules, 178–89
Five Minute Phobia Cure, 23
five point acupuncture, 14

five point touch therapy
   birth of, 16–18
   evolution of, 194–95
   explanation of, 4–6
   using the protocols, 148–50
   vital energy and, 12–16
   See also case studies
fourth golden rule, 22, 136–37,
   184–86

Gall Bladder 8, 94, *94*
Gall Bladder 34, 53, *53*, 60–61,
   60–61, 71, *71*, 126–27, *127*
Gall Bladder 38, 103, *103*
Gall Bladder 44, 58, *58*
golden rules, 178–89
Goodheart, George, 26
Governing Vessel 23, 35, *35*, 43, *43*,
   49, *49*, 87, *87*, 127, *127*, 130,
   130
grief, 7
guilt, 182–84

hair loss, 173
hand washing, 137
hatred. *See* anger
Heart 9, 108, *108*
heat, 16
homesickness. *See* nostalgia
hyperactivity, 162
hyper-emotionality, 46–50,
   47–50
Hyper-emotionality Protocol, 134,
   146–47
hypersomnia, 162
hypochondria, 162

impotence, 125–28, *126–28*, 163
inattention, 163
infections, repetitive, 163–64
insomnia, 27, 164
inspiration, lack of, 165
intuition, 129–32, *129–32*

jitters, 165
Jitters Protocol, 145–46

Kidney 1, 38, *38*
Kidney 3, 98, *98*, 112, *112*, 127, *127*
Kidney 6, 117, *117*
kinesiology, 23–26, *24*, *25*

Large Intestine 4, 33–34, *34*, 43, *43*,
   67, *67*, 72, *72*, 92, *92*, 102, *102*
Large Intestine 14, 29–30, *30*
lateral, 20
letting go, 165
libido, 125–28, *126–28*, 163, 165
Liver 2, 53, *53*, 82, *82*, 102, *102*
Liver 8, 125–26, *126*
loss, 165–66
love sickness, 166
lower back pain, 166
Lung 2, 49, *49*
Lung 7, 29, *29*, 34–35, *35*, 44, *44*,
   81–82, *82*, 88, *88*, 112–13,
   113
Lung 9, 107, *107*

medial, 20
mental challenges, 26
migraines, 166–67
mistakes, 182–84

morbid ideas, 27

muscle testing, *24, 25*

nadis, 13

nail-biting, 167

neck tightness, 167

needles, 16

negativity, 15, 32–36, *33–36,* 184–86, 191–92

neutral shields, 22, 136–37, 184–86

new environments, adapting, 168

nightmares, 167–68

night terrors, 168

nostalgia, 168–69

now, living in, 187–89

obesity, 169

Obesity Protocol, 146–47

Obsession Protocol, 143–46

obsessions, 42–45, *42–45,* 169, 175

overwork, 169

panic, 10–12, 37–41, *38–41,* 169

Panic Protocol, 141–43, 158

patches, 16–17

perfectionism, 170

Pericardium 6, 46–47, *47,* 56, *56,* 89, *89*

phobias, 37, 170

physical challenges, 26

points

application of technique, 21–22

locating, 19–21

See also specific points

positive energy, 193

prayer, 134

premature ejaculation, 170–71

premenstrual syndrome, 171

present, 187–89

"printed circuits," 4–5

proximal, 20

psoriasis, 172

psycho-bio-acupressure (PBA), 194–95

birth of, 16–18

explanation of, 4–6

using the protocols, 148–50

vital energy and, 12–16

See also case studies

psychosomatic reactions, 172–73

public speaking, 145–46

Rediscovering Real Medicine, 23, 140

Rescue Remedy, 135, 153

sacral plexus, 115–19, *116–19*

Salomé, Jacques, 105

scalp diseases, 173

scars, removing from energetic system, 51–55, *52–55*

second golden rule, 180–82

self-deprecation, 173

self-sabotage, 23–25

skin problems, 81–84, *82–84,* 85–90, *87–90,* 91–95, *91–95*

Small Intestine 8, 48, *48,* 98, *98*

solar plexus, 120–24, *121–24*

spasmophilia, 174

Special Point, 34, *34,* 57, *57,* 70–71, *71,* 73, *73,* 79, *79,* 107, *107,* 116, *116,* 121, *121*

Spleen 1, 28, *28,* 40, *40*

Spleen 4, 65–66, *66*

Spleen 6, 32–33, *33*, 54, *54*, 61, *61*, 72, *72*, 91, *91*, 99, *99*, 103, *103*, 109, *109*, 118, *118*, 121, *121*, 130, *130*

Spleen 10, 52, *52*, 58, *58*, 66, *66*, 126, *126*

Spleen 14, 78, *78*

Spleen 21, 111, *111*

stammering, 174

stimulation, 16

Stomach 7, 93, *93*

Stomach 25, 101, *101*

Stomach 36, 44, *44*, 62–63, *63*, 67, *67*, 79, *79*, 83, *83*, 99, *99*, 113, *113*, 116, *116*, 122, *122*, 131, *131*

Stomach 41, 108, *108*

stomach ulcers, 174

stories, 180–82

stress, 174, 179–80

suppressed anger, 70–74, *71–74*

symbolic objects, 105–6

third golden rule, 182–84

thoughts, 15, 25, 178

thyroid function, 105–10, *107–10*

tics, 175

tonsillitis, 175

trichotillomania, 176

Triple Heater 5, 39–40, *40*, 47, *47*, 62, *62*, 78, *78*, 82, *82*, 88, *88*, 123, *123*

Triple Heater 10, 83, *83*

Triple Heater 15, 28–29, *29*

ulcers, 174

uprooting, 176–77

Urinary Bladder 2, 57, *57*, 63, *63*, 92, *92*, 117, *117*, 122, *122*

Urinary Bladder 62, 54, *54*

Urinary Bladder 64, 87, *87*, 97, *97*

Urinary Bladder 67, 38, *38*, 68, *68*, 131, *131*

vaginal mycosis, 163–64, 177

ventral, 20

Véret, Patrick, 14, 23, 194–95

vibration, restoring fundamental, 56–59, *56–59*

vital energy, 12–16

watches, 22

yang, 13

yin, 13

yin/yang balance, 65–69, *66–69*